Thinking Politically about HIV

AIDS has a unique political history. As fears grew of a global pandemic on the scale of AIDS in sub-Saharan Africa, AIDS was briefly treated as an issue of high politics in the international arena and generated significant resources for country programmes. That initial commitment is now declining, and if AIDS is to maintain its visibility and contribution to global solidarity, human rights and dignity, its politics will have to evolve to reflect the profound geo-political, economic and social transformations underway today.

This volume brings together leading scholars from a variety of disciplines who work at the intersection of politics and HIV. They reflect on the lessons learned from the past thirty years of the politics of AIDS and how political science, writ large, can further contribute to the understanding and practice of political mobilization around AIDS. Through case studies and analysis, new insights into identity politics and social movements in countries as diverse as Brazil, Switzerland, Vietnam and Zambia are offered alongside new approaches to understanding the determinants and incentives which generate political will and commitment.

This book was published as a special issue of *Contemporary Politics*.

Kent Buse, PhD, is a political economist with a focus on health policy analysis. He is currently Chief of Political Affairs and Strategy at UNAIDS. He has taught at Yale University and at the London School of Hygiene and Tropical Medicine and has worked with a range of international organizations.

Dennis Altman is a political scientist who has written a number of key books on sexuality, HIV and AIDS, and Australian politics. He was President of the AIDS Society of Asia and the Pacific (2001-2005), and a member of the Governing Council of the International AIDS Society (2004-2012).

"In my experience as Head of India's AIDS programme during its intense phase, and later as Regional Director of UNAIDS in Asia Pacific, I have seen how politics plays a major defining role in AIDS responses in Asia Pacific countries ... As Buse and colleagues outline in this welcome collection, if we want to provide services to men who have sex with men, trans-genders, drug users and sex workers, every decision is a difficult political decision" - *Dr J.V.R. Prasada Rao, UN Secretary-General Special Envoy for AIDS*

"Whenever we have made progress on AIDS it was because of good politics. Whenever there was no progress, it was because of bad politics. This book provides unique analyses on the political forces and power relations that shaped the global AIDS response and provides critical lessons to shape the future" - *Professor Peter Piot, Director, London School of Hygiene and Tropical Medicine, UK*

"A judicious reminder that what is written, said, thought and done about the global AIDS crisis may no longer provide a self-assured basis upon which to construct future policy" - *Professor Nana Poku, Dean, School of Social and International Studies, Bradford University, UK*

"In this outstanding collection of essays, Buse, Altman and colleagues draw lessons from a thirty year struggle and make a timely call for paradigm shift in the global AIDS response" - *John Ferguson Professorial Chair of African Studies, Bradford University, UK*

Thinking Politically about HIV

Edited by
Kent Buse and Dennis Altman

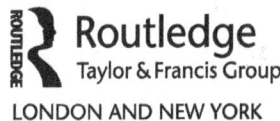

LONDON AND NEW YORK

First published 2014 by Routledge

2 Park Square, Milton Park, Abingdon, Oxfordshire OX14 4RN
711 Third Avenue, New York, NY 10017

Routledge is an imprint of the Taylor & Francis Group, an informa business

First issued in paperback 2018

Copyright © 2014 Taylor & Francis

This book is a reproduction of *Contemporary Politics*, vol. 18, issue 2. The Publisher requests to those authors who may be citing this book to state, also, the bibliographical details of the special issue on which the book was based.

All rights reserved. No part of this book may be reprinted or reproduced or utilised in any form or by any electronic, mechanical, or other means, now known or hereafter invented, including photocopying and recording, or in any information storage or retrieval system, without permission in writing from the publishers.

Notice:
Product or corporate names may be trademarks or registered trademarks, and are used only for identification and explanation without intent to infringe.

British Library Cataloguing in Publication Data
A catalogue record for this book is available from the British Library

ISBN13: 978-0-415-82554-2 (hbk)
ISBN13: 978-1-138-38326-5 (pbk)

Typeset in Times New Roman
by Taylor & Francis Books

Publisher's Note
The publisher would like to make readers aware that the chapters in this book may be referred to as articles as they are identical to the articles published in the special issue. The publisher accepts responsibility for any inconsistencies that may have arisen in the course of preparing this volume for print.

Contents

Citation Information vii
Notes on Contributors ix

1. Thinking politically about HIV: political analysis and action in response to AIDS
   Dennis Altman and Kent Buse 1

2. Political science(s) and HIV: a critical analysis
   Nathan A. Paxton 15

3. Descriptive representation and AIDS policy in South Africa
   Evan S. Lieberman 30

4. Public opinion as leadership disincentive: exploring a governance dilemma in the AIDS response in Africa
   Per Strand 48

5. Building capacities and producing citizens: the biopolitics of HIV prevention in Brazil
   Rafael de la Dehesa and Ananya Mukherjea 60

6. Constitution, diversification and normalization of a health problem: organizing the fight against AIDS in Switzerland (1984–2005)
   Michael Voegtli and Olivier Fillieule 74

7. AIDS mobilisation in Zambia and Vietnam: explaining the differences
   Amy S. Patterson and David Stephens 87

8. China's evolving AIDS policy: the influence of global norms and transnational non-governmental organizations
   Joan Kaufman 99

9. Lessons from the rise and fall of the military AIDS hypothesis: politics, evidence and persuasion
   Michael O'Keefe 113

10. AIDS hyper-epidemics and social resilience: theorising the political
    Pieter Fourie and Maj-Lis Follér 128

Index 143

Citation Information

The chapters in this book were originally published in *Contemporary Politics*, volume 18, issue 4 (June 2012). When citing this material, please use the original page numbering for each article, as follows:

Chapter 1
Thinking politically about HIV: political analysis and action in response to AIDS
Dennis Altman and Kent Buse
Contemporary Politics, volume 18, issue 4 (June 2012) pp. 127-140

Chapter 2
Political science(s) and HIV: a critical analysis
Nathan A. Paxton
Contemporary Politics, volume 18, issue 4 (June 2012) pp. 141-155

Chapter 3
Descriptive representation and AIDS policy in South Africa
Evan S. Lieberman
Contemporary Politics, volume 18, issue 4 (June 2012) pp. 156-173

Chapter 4
Public opinion as leadership disincentive: exploring a governance dilemma in the AIDS response in Africa
Per Strand
Contemporary Politics, volume 18, issue 4 (June 2012) pp. 174-185

Chapter 5
Building capacities and producing citizens: the biopolitics of HIV prevention in Brazil
Rafael de la Dehesa and Ananya Mukherjea
Contemporary Politics, volume 18, issue 4 (June 2012) pp. 186-199

Chapter 6
Constitution, diversification and normalization of a health problem: organizing the fight against AIDS in Switzerland (1984–2005)
Michael Voegtli and Olivier Fillieule
Contemporary Politics, volume 18, issue 4 (June 2012) pp. 200-212

CITATION INFORMATION

Chapter 7
AIDS mobilisation in Zambia and Vietnam: explaining the differences
Amy S. Patterson and David Stephens
Contemporary Politics, volume 18, issue 4 (June 2012) pp. 213-224

Chapter 8
China's evolving AIDS policy: the influence of global norms and transnational non-governmental organizations
Joan Kaufman
Contemporary Politics, volume 18, issue 4 (June 2012) pp. 225-238

Chapter 9
Lessons from the rise and fall of the military AIDS hypothesis: politics, evidence and persuasion
Michael O'Keefe
Contemporary Politics, volume 18, issue 4 (June 2012) pp. 239-253

Chapter 10
AIDS hyper-epidemics and social resilience: theorising the political
Pieter Fourie and Maj-Lis Follér
Contemporary Politics, volume 18, issue 4 (June 2012) pp. 254-268

Notes on Contributors

Dennis Altman is Professor and Director of the Institute for Human Security, La Trobe University, Melbourne, Australia

Kent Buse is Chief of Political Affairs and Strategy, UNAIDS, Geneva, Switzerland

Rafael de la Dehesa is Associate Professor in Sociology at City University of New York, USA

Olivier Fillieule is Professor of Political Sociology at Lausanne University, Switzerland

Maj-Lis Follér is Professor at the Institute for Global Studies at Gothenburg University, Sweden

Pieter Fourie is Professor of Politics at Stellenbosch University, South Africa

Joan Kaufman is Director of Columbia University's Global Center/East Asia, Beijing, China

Evan S. Lieberman is Professor of Politics at Princeton University, USA

Ananya Mukherjea is Associate Professor of Sociology at City University of New York, USA

Michael O'Keefe is Senior Lecturer in International Relations at La Trobe University, Melbourne, Australia

Amy S. Patterson is Professor in the Department of Political Science, University of the South, USA

Nathan A. Paxton is a Research Fellow at the School of International Service, American University, Washington DC, USA

David Stephens is Chief of Party in the USAID Pathways for Participation Project, Vietnam

Per Strand is Research Associate at the University of Cape Town and M&E Manager at Star for Life, South Africa

Michael Voegtli is Visiting Professor at Universidad Autónoma Metropolitana, Mexico City, Mexico

Thinking politically about HIV: political analysis and action in response to AIDS

Dennis Altman and Kent Buse

AIDS has a uniquely political history. Its early association with stigmatised homosexual behaviour and more liberating gay identity activism set the precedent for highly effective mobilisation. The results were unparalleled in global health. AIDS was briefly treated as high politics and attracted increased funds to achieve the ambitious goal of universal access to HIV prevention and treatment. If AIDS is to maintain its visibility and contribution to global solidarity, human rights and dignity, its politics must evolve to reflect the profound geo-political, economic and social transformations currently underway. 'Thinking politically about HIV', an initiative of UNAIDS and the International AIDS Society, was convened in recognition of the need to better understand these politics and consider how the political sciences can further engage. This paper, and the edited volume it introduces, provides some insights into the *Thinking Politically* discussions as well as the wider scholarship on the challenges facing the AIDS response. The authors argue that while mainstream political science has largely ignored the epidemic, other disciplines and traditions provide rich accounts of the exceptional response. Given the changing context, the authors present an agenda of practically oriented, politically informed research to identify the levers that can be used to maintain the viability of the response.

One of us, writing about AIDS in the early 1980s, termed it 'the most political of diseases'. The connection of AIDS to largely stigmatised personal behaviours set it apart from other infectious diseases, and ensured it would involve affected communities politically in ways that have few, if any, precedents. While the control of sexually transmitted infections has long been a significant concern of governments, this concern was largely confined to their control in the uniformed service rather than through universal surveillance and services. The early debates within the USA and other western countries foreshadowed issues of stigma, rights and social justice that were not matched in the history of other communicable illnesses, making for what has become known as 'AIDS exceptionalism'. Thirty years after the syndrome was recognised and then named, AIDS continues to be the subject of political debate of a sort rarely experienced around a disease.

1. Political analysis of HIV and AIDS

We assume that the subjects of political analysis are the authoritative allocation of resources, or as Harold Lasswell memorably put it in a foundation text of contemporary political science: 'who gets what, when and how' (Lasswell 1936). The earliest political analyses of the epidemic (e.g. Patton 1985, Altman 1986, Watney 1986, Crimp 1988) grew directly out of the experience of western gay movements, who were the primary stakeholders in the first few years. Because of the link to communities where there already existed an understanding that 'the personal is political', from its inception AIDS saw ongoing challenges to the usual dominance of biomedical expertise, leading to the creation of new forms of involvement in policy-making by those most touched by the epidemic.

It is common for speakers at international AIDS conferences to talk of the importance of politics, particularly the need for political will, while ignoring the need for sustained and careful political analysis. Indeed political science as a discipline has been barely represented at these conferences, where what social science is presented tends to be behavioural, and seen as relevant in so far as it duplicates the methodologies of biomedicine (or affords biomedicine access to policy makers). Scientists quite often conflate social, cultural and political analysis with advocacy. The XIX International AIDS Conference in Washington, DC, this year, for example, devotes a research track to 'social science, human rights and political science', as if human rights were itself a discipline rather than a particular set of values and principles that are equally relevant to all disciplines represented in the Conference programme (Kippax and Holt 2009). What IS worthy of political analysis is the ways in which AIDS has been the catalyst in producing new links between health and human rights, links which are themselves contentious and the subject of political debate (Gruskin *et al.* 2007).

There are certain terms, common to political science, which are used a great deal in 'AIDS-speak' – civil society, political commitment, leadership, social movements, etc. – which have a long and complex history of analysis that is largely ignored by those invoking these concepts. Our experience is that 'civil society', for example, is commonly used to describe whichever assortment of 'community organisations' [itself a term deserving of analysis] is able to be present in the room when the phrase is used as opposed to in the Gramscian sense of creating a political space for critical debate between citizens and state. As some of the papers in this issue demonstrate (e.g. Lieberman), there is a dearth of analytic thinking about 'political commitment' and 'political will', despite the frequency with which these terms are used in the AIDS response. After all, what could suggest greater 'commitment' than the image of President Mbeki surfing the Internet late into the night to find evidence against the HIV-AIDS hypothesis, and what could be less constructive as a response? Even weak governments have the power to block, to hinder and to put obstacles in the way of community organisations and healthcare workers who are trying to respond to the needs of people living with HIV or at risk of exposure through sex work, their sexuality or needle use, and governments (and other interest/value groups) are often good at using rhetoric to cloak their real intentions and abilities. One example is the number of countries whose national HIV plans talk about outreach to marginalised populations while in practice retaining punitive laws, police harassment and punishment of those very populations.

Given the political nature of the disease, the extraordinary political mobilisation by people living with and most affected by HIV and the consequent transformations achieved by these communities in relation to health service delivery, resource mobilisation, governance and legislation, it seems to us that there is a strong case for greater political analysis of the AIDS response. Identity politics, transnational social movement formation, strategic litigation and other tactics for political change are not unique to the AIDS response, but have been distinctive and exercised in a manner unusual in global health. Indeed, some have argued that the response has been too successful and that resources mobilised for AIDS ought to be channelled to diseases that do not enjoy the same level of support and attention. Given that half of those who need treatment cannot access it and that two people acquire HIV for every person who successfully initiates treatment, there remains a pressing need for continued political mobilisation, but this demands an appreciation and analysis of the fast changing political and financial environment, and hence demands new and different political responses.

2. The 'thinking politically about HIV' initiative

Recognising the need for more rigorous and analytic thinking about the political dimensions of HIV, the International AIDS Society (IAS) and Joint United Nations Programme on HIV/AIDS (UNAIDS) embarked upon an initiative to build better links between researchers in the political sciences [including international relations and development studies] and those working directly in AIDS policy and programming.

The origins of the initiative date back to a meeting convened by the IAS in Cape Town, South Africa, in 2009, where the absence of good political analysis was noted as a significant gap in the AIDS research agenda. The need to enhance analysis is reflected in both the IAS Strategic Plan (2010–2014) and UNAIDS current leadership, Mission and Strategy (2011–2015). As representatives of the two sponsoring organisations – Altman from IAS and Buse from UNAIDS – we convened an advisory group which met in Vienna during the 2010 XVIII International AIDS Conference, and with considerable assistance from the UNAIDS regional office in Bangkok convened an international workshop there in April 2011.

The papers in this collection are to some extent a product of that workshop, which brought together political scientists and practitioners, both at government and community level, from a range of countries. Inevitably the meeting was not as geographically diverse as we would have liked, but it did allow for some remarkable interchanges between senior political figures, academics and community activists, focusing on how best to develop analysis that was both conceptually rich and of practical use to people working on programmes and advocacy. Two strands of discussion stand out. The first, dominated by political figures, focused on the extent to which politicians lead or follow – that is; follow the political incentives emanating from the public, media and advocacy groups. The second was the challenge posed by practitioners to the academic community who were seen as failing to provide much convincing theory or to adapt the findings of research into practical tools to guide action to engage more effectively in the political arena. The themes of that workshop led onto a panel at the International Conference on AIDS in Asia and the Pacific, the regional AIDS Conference for Asia and the Pacific, in Busan, South Korea, in August 2011, and to events at the SAHARA Conference in South Africa in December that year.

3. The political achievements of AIDS activism

The political history of the epidemic over the past three decades has witnessed some remarkable successes. HIV has been placed on the international agenda, with a specific UN programme, UNAIDS, created to coordinate the responses of different parts of the UN system to HIV, to inspire and inform the global response as well as to provide support to countries. The epidemic was the subject of a special meeting of the United Nations Security Council (2000) and three special sessions of the General Assembly (2001, 2006, 2011). AIDS is specifically mentioned in the millennium development goals (MDGs), and the creation of the Global Fund to Fight AIDS, Tuberculosis and Malaria has ensured considerable resources flow towards prevention and treatment. Set up in 2002, by 2011 the Global Fund had approved more than US$22 billion in grants, although, as is discussed later, spending is now slowing markedly.

In some parts of the world, HIV has opened up space for discussion of sexuality and, to a lesser extent, drug use in quite unprecedented ways, and has meant considerable support for organisation and advocacy amongst marginalised and stigmatised populations (Kane 1998, Kempadoo and Doezema 1998, Altman 2001). HIV has changed attitudes of health care providers, and has created new paradigms of relationships between practitioners and patients that have affected other significant diseases. In short, AIDS altered existing balances of power.

The clinical discovery of what would become known as HIV was first noted amongst homosexual men in the USA, although earlier cases clearly existed in Africa. This would establish a framework that remains even today – where discourses on AIDS are dominated by the particular political demands and stigma that marked its early history in the USA. In the USA, as in other western countries, the early response to the epidemic was led by gay community organisations in a remarkable example of mobilisation, often without much support from governments. In many developing countries gay movements would develop in large part because of the challenge of the new epidemic, just as AIDS led to a certain amount of organisation among sex workers and drug users (e.g. Altman 1994, Andriote 1999, de la Dehasa and Mukherjea, 2012, Fillieule and Voegtil, 2012).

As it became clear that the epidemic existed far beyond western gay communities, the World Health Organisation established the first international programme under the leadership of Jonathan Mann. By the mid-1990s, this programme was replaced by UNAIDS. The USA was slow to recognise the extent of the global epidemic, but particularly under the administration of George W. Bush it came to place considerable emphasis on providing assistance for both treatment and prevention, even if, in the latter case, in ways consistent with a particular moralistic stance. Indeed under Bush some of the most ardent proponents of international support for HIV programmes came from the religious right, who came to see it as a major moral imperative (Altman 2010).

Today roughly half of all global resources available to combat HIV come from the USA. The politics of AIDS are to some extent shaped by American responses, as in the development of a politics that stresses the empowerment of those who are infected and affected. This is reflected in international rhetoric [not always borne out in practice] around 'the greater involvement of people with AIDS'. Outside sub-Saharan Africa, AIDS remains closely associated with stigmatised behaviours – commercial and homosexual sex; injecting drug use – and the epidemic has greatly strengthened organising amongst groups who practise such behaviour. Nonetheless, not all those who engage in potentially risky behaviour will feel impelled to organise: there is virtually no sense of community amongst men who buy sex, for example.

The AIDS world is dominated by the politics of experience: demand for representation sometimes overshadows demand for expertise. But experience without analysis is as poor a guide for action as analysis without experience. And the emphasis on identity politics, while often empowering, can also elide the reality that most people who engage in stigmatised and possibly dangerous behaviours do so without any sense of identity. Inevitably the politics of AIDS are plagued by unresolved questions about representation and voice, which are not sufficiently discussed.

These elements of the AIDS response would make for strange bed-fellows but also deliver remarkable results. Treatment access in sub-Saharan Africa is illustrative. As noted, the US conservative right rallied around the imagery of suffering, innocent children (and their mothers) and the opportunity to export precepts of morality and expand church membership. Progressive activists and human rights campaigners developed transnational coalitions, which put pressure on donors, drug companies, governments and international trade regimes for treatment access. Drug companies initially responded with litigation but this strategy was quickly replaced with corporate social responsibility schemes including drug donations and tiered pricing. The volte-face by drug makers was prompted in part by public attitudes but also by the calculus that donors would more or less subsidise the production costs of treatment. For their part, donors saw in treatment programmes an ability to count the number of people they would put on treatment (and lives saved) – this was as appealing as it was easy to explain to sceptical tax payers impatient with vague and remote development cooperation initiatives. The particular confluence of political incentives was unique to treatment access, but what next?

4. Current challenges facing the AIDS response

Put bluntly, the current challenge facing those who advocate for AIDS programmes is that investment needs are increasing, just at a time when global financial commitments to the response are declining.

As the global impact of AIDS became more evident in the 1990s, the expectation was that western countries, lead by the USA, should lead and fund much of the response. The well-publicised Security Council and General Assembly sessions on AIDS in 2001 were followed by increasing attention from the G-8, the group of the world's leading first world economies who at its Gleneagles summit in 2005 pledged universal access to HIV drugs in Africa by 2010, as well as a doubling of aid overall to the continent. A number of factors came together to achieve these goals, in particular the mobilisation of extensive civil society networks through the Make Poverty History movement, and the personal commitment of the host country, Britain, under Tony Blair, strongly supported by Presidents Bush and Chirac. That year may well have marked the high point of the rich world's concern for African development in general, and HIV in particular: this particular confluence of interests may never be repeated.

The work at Gleneagles was facilitated by the adoption by the UN in 2000 of the MDGs, which came to form the basic 'global operating framework for development'. The sixth MDG specifies: Target 6A: Have halted by 2015 and begun to reverse the spread of HIV/AIDS; and Target 6B: Achieve, by 2010, universal access to treatment for HIV/AIDS for all those who need it. Additional MDGs, particularly those relating to the empowerment of women, reduction of child mortality and improving maternal health, are closely related. The MDGs will expire in 2015, and discussions have begun about what goals might be set by international community (including donors) in a post-MDG world. There is no reason to assume that a future set of international priorities will include HIV. There is an urgent need to reflect on how the connections between human rights and health as well as social justice and equity, that have been the hallmarks of the AIDS response, might be enshrined in a post-MDG declaration.

Six years after Gleneagles the world is a very different place. Two aspects in particular are relevant to this discussion: declining concern with AIDS globally and significant shifts in the balance of economic and cultural power.

It is no longer possible to suggest that HIV is a global pandemic that will see the horrific figures from southern and eastern Africa reached in other parts of the world. Even in Papua New Guinea, probably the worst affected country in the Asia/Pacific region, HIV prevalence is less than a tenth of that in many African countries. Yet less than a decade ago the conservative scholar Nicholas Eberstadt warned of a major pandemic in Eurasia that 'will alter the economic potential of the region's major states and the global balance of power' (Eberstadt 2002). This did not occur, and the tragedy of AIDS today is that it is unequally affecting the most vulnerable and marginalised, in terms of geography, gender and behaviour, and it is increasingly difficult to persuade most people that it is a global priority on the same level as climate change, food and water shortages, and the persistence of fragile and unstable states across many parts of the world. It would appear that even across much of sub-Saharan Africa, public opinion places many other issues ahead of HIV (see Strand, 2012).

In the same way simplistic arguments that HIV would be spread through a breakdown of security, alarmist stories about the very high rate of HIV amongst soldiers and peace-keepers have been largely discredited by careful research (see the summary of the evidence in reviews produced by the de Waal *et al.*, 2010 as well as O'Keefe, 2012). But this does not mean that the dislocations due to conflict do not increase vulnerability to infection while making it more difficult to establish effective programmes or even provide basic information and services. The long-term impact of growing needle use and commercial sex in parts of the world ravaged by conflict – think of the huge population shifts across Iraq, Afghanistan and Pakistan over the past decade – are likely to lead to increasing HIV infection, and once a number of people are infected the epidemic has always the potential to escalate rapidly.

The political reality is that AIDS cried wolf too often, and the more dire warnings have failed to materialise. In most parts of the world, AIDS is not a security or development crisis, and the perception that the response has received too much attention and funding is growing. It is absolutely true, as the eminent group who prepared the *AIDS 2031 Report* have argued, that: 'Closing the looming funding gap for AIDS would require only about 1% of annual global spending on armaments' (Aids2031 2010). In the same way that the gap could be plugged with just 1.5% of the yield of the financial transactions tax promoted by a number of European governments, as well as numerous economists and activists. Yet in the absence of new generalised epidemics affecting large parts of the adult population, as is true across south and eastern Africa, such appeals will fall on deaf ears. When there were plausible arguments that HIV threatened political and military stability in significant countries it shot to the top of international attention. It is hardly surprising that as these fears have diminished so has interest in the epidemic lagged.

It is a further tragedy that as the biomedical means to control HIV are increasingly viable, the resources to ensure access to them are likely to further decrease, which suggests the imperative to concentrate resources on the most cost-effective prevention programmes (Schwartländer *et al.* 2011). Not only are traditional donor countries cutting back on their contributions to international development assistance, they are doing so within a world in which political and economic power continues to shift rapidly. The G-8 still meets, but it has been essentially replaced by the G-20 as the steering group of major economies. Given that the G-20 includes several countries with significant epidemics, most notably South Africa, and others with strong commitment to universal access, in particular Brazil and China, one might expect the G-20 to take a position of leadership on global HIV efforts. Both South Africa and Brazil are core countries in emerging new partnerships linking a number of middle-income countries with increasing global political and economic influence. The G-20 and the BRICS states (Brazil, Russia, India, China, South Africa) may push for greater access to therapeutic drugs and greater support for generics, but they are unlikely to view HIV as a major concern without significant prompting. Moreover, the G-8 was able to mobilise donor countries in ways that the G-20 is unlikely to do.

In part this is because the shifts in global power are creating new nationalisms and challenging western norms of individualistic human rights. Countries such as China, Korea and the Gulf states, which are becoming more important as donors to the developing world, are more committed to protecting state sovereignty and far less likely to demand basic human rights than more traditional western donor countries. While we see increasing pressure from western countries around issues such as human rights and protection of confidentiality – both the UK and USA recently announced they would consider aid funding decisions in the context of the human rights record of recipients, including sexual rights – such pressures are likely to be undermined by donors for which these are not priorities (although Kaufman, 2012, argues that transnational NGOs can alter the perceived interests and norms of powerful states such as China). Good political analysis would not just deplore the decline of interest and resources in the

5. The failure of conventional political science

> A political scientist can do little more than what a journalist does: go to places where there appear to be interesting linkages between, say, land scarcity and violence, and see if causal relationships exist. From this, some useful ideas or theories might emerge. To call it science, though, is an overstatement. (Kaplan 1997)

The dominant paradigm of American political science, as the very name of the discipline suggests, is to quantify and to seek provable causal relationships between variables. This is difficult to do in many areas of political activity, and little in AIDS lends itself to such analysis. Indeed the dominant paradigms of political science are largely Anglo-American, and this is reflected in our problem in finding participants and authors in the *Thinking Politically* initiative from developing countries. This does not mean there is a lack of political analysis, only that it is not accessible through the same rubrics as in rich English-speaking countries.

Of course there are other traditions of political science – as the names 'sciences politiques' or 'Staatswissenschaft' should remind us – but increasingly academics who see themselves as belonging to the discipline feel pressure to publish in, and conform to, the norms of the American and British academic establishment.[1]

As Paxton (2012) discusses, mainstream political science, at least in Anglo-American countries, has not been much interested in the politics of the epidemic. Of course some political scientists have done important work on HIV, including the group of scholars in international relations who have analysed the implications of positioning HIV as a security threat. Paxton's paper describes a number of the studies that do exist, and we are aware of a growing number of doctoral theses being written. The three of us share a limited knowledge of the literature in other languages, though we note that there are a number of studies on the politics of HIV in French, Portuguese and Spanish.

The absence of much political science analysis of the epidemic is particularly striking given the high priority placed on HIV by the second Bush administration, the volume of resources devoted to the US PEPFAR programme[2] as well as the tendency of many of those involved to claim 'AIDS exceptionalism', namely that it remains fundamentally different to other public health issues (e.g. Smith and Whiteside 2010). Indeed, HIV has been more amenable to analysis in cognate disciplines, such as public policy, international relations and development studies. There is a growing literature in public health that deals with HIV, sometimes drawing on key political concepts to do so (e.g. Brown and Labonte 2011).

Politically oriented analysis of the AIDS response has come from other disciplines, notably history, anthropology and sociology, where a number of scholars have written careful studies of the impact of, and response to, the epidemic (e.g. Berridge and Strong 1993, Epstein 1996, Carrillo 2002, Sendziuk 2003, Fassin 2007). Conventional political science ignores both the idea that 'the personal is political' and the central importance of culture [and religion] – which anthropology brings to bear on the subject.

But analysis, too, has often come from other traditions, notably from journalists and from people writing out of their experiences at a community level (e.g. Frasca 2005, Geffen 2010). The best-known book from the early history of the epidemic is Randy Shilts' *And the Band Played on*, written by someone who was deeply involved as both a reporter in San Francisco and a member of the most affected community (Shilts 1987). While Shilts was criticised for poor epidemiology and his invention of a mythical 'Patient Zero', the book had a large readership and continues to be influential. A more dispassionate journalistic analysis has come from

Helen Epstein who has carefully analysed the Ugandan response to the epidemic (Epstein 2007), just as Michael Specter has done for Russia in the *New Yorker* (Specter 2004). In much of Asia the most sophisticated analysis of the epidemic has come from journalists rather than academics, and of course a great deal of analysis is contained, if only implicitly, in reports written for governments and international agencies.

Nor should we ignore the considerable creative literature that has emanated from the experience of the epidemic, which chronicles in quite remarkable ways how the epidemic has impacted upon particular groups and societies. While most literary reflections tend to concentrate on personal experience, often to the exclusion of larger social and political contexts, they remain an interesting insight into the ongoing and sometimes indirect ravages of the epidemic. At their best theatre, novels and film can illuminate and mobilise. Two plays, Larry Kramer's *The Normal Heart* (1985) and Tony Kushner's *Angels in America* (1993), provide powerful examples of this. While much of the literary response has come from western gay writers there is some writing, particularly from Africa, which illuminates the experiences of HIV in ways not always possible through academic writing (e.g. Dow 2000, Steinberg 2008).

One of the most obvious gaps in the literature of AIDS is serious analysis of the role played by 'culture, religion and tradition' in preventing honest discussion of the behaviours that can lead to transmission of HIV, even though in many parts of the world this remains a significant barrier to effective prevention efforts. Hypocrisy, said, Francois de La Rochefoucauld, is the homage which vice pays to virtue, and AIDS is an arena replete with such hypocrisies. This might provide an interesting framework for a political analysis of the response to the epidemic, but it is not one likely to be used by academic political scientists.

Some of the concepts and theories of political science have been drawn upon to inform the broad rubric of policy studies. The policy literature on HIV is eclectic and unified simply in describing the ideas, institutions and interests, and sometimes their interactions, which appear to be associated with agenda setting, policy formulation or implementation. There is some work on western countries, yet more recently most research has focused on Brazil, Senegal, Thailand and Uganda (due to early and positive policy change) and South Africa (due to the highly contested nature of the policy response) with a limited number of comparative works (Schneider and Stein 2001, Schneider 2002, Allen and Heald 2004, Parkhurst and Lush 2004, Putzel 2004, 2006, Berkman *et al.* 2005, Butler 2005, Gauri and Lieberman 2006, Heald 2006, Bor 2007, Lieberman 2007). Others have looked at how to improve the political palatability of evidence-informed policies in a prospective manner (e.g. Buse *et al.* 2009) as well as how to manage researcher-policy-community relationships to ensure better evidence-informed and relevant policy for marginalised groups (Hawkes *et al.*, 2012).

6. An agenda for future research

We make no pretence that the collection in this volume does little more than open up some areas for reflection, and is limited geographically, linguistically and in terms of subject matter. Some themes do however run through the papers: a concern with governmentality, in its broadest sense; with civil society; and with social movements. Discussions over the course of the *Thinking Politically* initiative revealed a number of areas that deserve further conceptualisation and research.

The likely impacts of changes in the global environment on the politics of AIDS responses are of intrinsic and instrumental importance. In 2010 external finance for the response flat-lined for the first time – this in the context of programmes that, particularly in Africa, are heavily dependent on donor funds. Moreover, over the past five years a number of countries have moved from being defined as 'low-' to 'middle-income' – where a billion poor people now reside – and thus are no longer eligible for assistance from some aid sources. Many African economies are surging and BRICS countries are assuming greater responsibility for their own AIDS responses as well as more pronounced regional and global donorship roles. In short, trends in foreign assistance are shifting rapidly. The rise of non-traditional donors may curtail the support that some marginalised groups can expect to receive – a trend that may be reinforced in North Africa with the rise of Islamic-oriented, democratic regimes. New ways of addressing culturally sensitive issues need to be found. Another aspect of the changing global environment concerns the pharmaceutical sector. Implementation of the TRIPS as well as 'TRIPS+' agreements and restructuring of the generics industry may mean that the factors that led to the relative affordability of first line ARVs may not hold in so far as second and third line regimens are concerned. These and other global trends suggest very different politics for AIDS in the coming decade.

The changing linkages between AIDS and other issues of international development and human security deserve ongoing analysis. There is a small body of work that seeks to link concerns about climate change to HIV, and more on the connections to mass population movements, food and water, security, etc. (McMichael 2009). Fourie and Follér (2012) creatively employ theorising from the natural sciences to examine the political resilience of societies to the long-wave event that is AIDS. Nonetheless, the fact remains that surprisingly little has been written about the interconnection of HIV and the other priorities of the MDGs, even though this may well be crucial in discussions concerning the post-2015 development framework.

Much can be learned from a comparative study of national (and sometimes state or provincial) AIDS responses, in particular a better understanding of the specific factors that support or hinder particular approaches to HIV. There is little analysis of the politics that affect, for example, laws and policing of drug use and needle exchange, which vary enormously, often in ways that are not easily predictable (e.g. comparatively progressive policies in Malaysia and Iran, but increasingly restrictive ones in Russia and Uzbekistan). And the same holds true of the (de)criminalisation of sex workers and/or their clients across countries as well as how countries address sexuality education or condom access. And this need not involve new empirical research. Paxton's (2012) review of the literature reveals a number of case studies of the politics of AIDS in different contexts, suggesting the potential for rigorous synthesis work.

The political dimensions of religious and cultural barriers to prevention remain critical to the progression of the epidemic. In many countries, religious leaders have spearheaded opposition to promotion of condoms and safe sex education. Christian and Islamic fundamentalist groups are increasingly lobbying governments and the UN to promote socially conservative family norms as well as cultural and religious values, which may impede universal access to HIV prevention and other services. For example, Family Watch International, a US-based advocacy group, has developed a sophisticated strategy to promote 'family values' and criminal laws against homosexuality, which involves providing support for conservative legislators in Africa while lobbying UN delegates in New York. Better understanding of how these groups work may support efforts to ensure their influence does not undermine evidence-informed programmes.

The role of media in framing agendas and policy alternatives as well as building public support in favour or against HIV programmes. Analysis suggests that press freedoms play a role in explaining political commitment to strong AIDS responses (e.g. Bor 2007). Others suggest that it is not freedoms *per se* but the relationship between policy makers and journalists (e.g. Lomax Cook et al. 1983) in line with Sabatier's advocacy coalition framework model (Sabatier 1988). This area of research would include the emerging role of social media, and its linkages with interest groups, in terms of movement and interest (values) formation, and how this plays out in political decision-making.

Social movements and identity politics have been central to government responses to HIV. There is a substantial academic literature on how certain vulnerable groups, most particularly homosexual men, have responded to the epidemic (Fillieule and Voegtil, 2012, De la Dehesa and Mukherjea, 2012). Much of this literature is ignored by activists, who rely heavily on official reports or advocacy documents, and are impatient with what they see as the unnecessary qualifications of academic theorising. The literature on other vulnerable groups is far smaller, and there are few good studies of attempts to create a sense of community and political empowerment amongst, say, sex workers or injectors (see Patterson and Stephens, 2012, in relation to intravenous drug users).[3] There is some interesting research on AIDS activism (e.g. Friedman and Mottiar 2004, Gould 2009), as well as some that points to the difficulties facing different minority groups organising for common cause (e.g. Kendall and Lopez-Uribe 2010) but there is need for much better analysis of how activism impacts upon policy making.

Further analysis of how the concepts of human rights are (and could be) deployed in relation to AIDS and other development challenges, for example gender. The development of the links between health and human rights is an important legacy of the growth of international responses to AIDS.[4] Yet, there is an urgent need to reconsider how useful the concept is in a rapidly changing global and resource environment. It is arguable that the western concept of human rights, with its considerable emphasis on the individual, is less applicable in societies with different concepts of community and privacy (e.g. de Waal 2003).

An examination of the institutions established by the AIDS world and how they evolve, or fail to, would be instructive both for the response and other issue areas. Parker (2011) has written an account of shifts in the global AIDS movement, but there is a need for ongoing studies of the ways in which UNAIDS, the Global Fund, UNITAID, the Bill and Melinda Gates Foundation as well as other financiers and governing bodies (e.g. UNODC) operate to influence policies and responses to HIV, both globally and nationally. While there are analyses of the Global Fund in the public health literature, they do not interrogate how the Fund is governed or makes decisions (e.g. Ooms *et al.* 2008). Similarly, although there have been calls to shut down UNAIDS (England 2008, 2011), these have not been informed by serious analysis of the value-added of the programme. Many of the institutions that constitute the AIDS architecture, including UNAIDS, the IAS and the International Council of AIDS Service Organisations, are now reaching adulthood. It is necessary to reassess their added-value, and whether or not their roles remain relevant as the larger environment itself changes. Similarly, as more NGOs evolve from advocacy to service provision functions [and do so as resources available to them diminish], can they maintain the tradition of challenging the status quo – from intellectual property regimes, to norms governing sexuality and gender – and if not, what are the implications for the progressive nature of the response? Ironically, activist organisations such as ACT UP or the Treatment Action Coalition in its early days were more likely to produce 'organic intellectuals' [i.e. people who combined activism with scholarship] than the more respectable and co-opted movements that have now become an integral part of the AIDS establishment. As someone, perhaps William Buckley, once observed: 'Every cause begins as a social movement, becomes an organisation, and ends up as a cabal'.

7. Politics as art rather than science

During discussions generated by the *Thinking Politically* initiative some discontent was expressed by practitioners about the lack of immediate practical application to the analyses presented by academics. Yet, as *The Economist* put it, 'there is political utility in thinking, for few things are more politically toxic than a lack of ideas' (The Economist 2011). Without an understanding of the broader political environment, whether global or national, programmes will not be effective, and without an ongoing analysis of wider trends, AIDS will decline in salience amongst all those but its immediate constituency. Clearly, we ought to embrace both *thinking* and *acting* politically.

While there exist plenty of off-the-shelf tools to aid practitioners in stakeholder analysis, as well as software variants, there is more to navigating politics than identifying stakeholder interests – action needs to be guided by consideration of context and issue- and institution-specific processes as well. Evidence suggests that collaborative action-research involving practitioners and researchers can open vistas to more relevant research and better-informed action (Nutely et al. 2007, Ward et al. 2009). Such partnership is admittedly difficult not only because of the impatience of practitioners and the incentives driving researchers, but also because it raises questions of legitimacy and introduces bias into the research process – although the latter can be addressed through practices of reflexivity, triangulation, etc.

But the challenge goes beyond the availability of tools and comes to the question of mindsets. For example, the experiences of HIV have infused much academic and non-academic writing on gender, sexuality and identity, but all too often this literature fails to connect with what practitioners read or consider. Thinking and acting politically requires a kind of openness and approach to enquiry – which is challenging to academics and practitioners alike.

Perhaps we should think of political analysis as we think of medicine, which necessarily combines objective science with subjective judgements, as each patient presents with a unique biological, environmental and psychological background. The search for general explanations are too often founded on the particulars, but at the same time can focus our attention on questions that too specific an analysis can miss. Despite the rather misleading term 'political science' it is important to remember that its models are fundamentally differently to those in the physical and biological sciences (Derman 2011).

Through the *Thinking Politically* initiative we have sought to marry the art and science of politics with the approaches of those working in the academie, those supporting programmes, and those in communities. We see ongoing value in more systematically bringing 'political animals' together in ways that biomed is much better at doing.

Acknowledgements

Thanks to our Advisory Committee, some of whom are represented in this volume. We are grateful to the reviewers of the papers in this volume, owe an intellectual debt to the participants at the Bangkok workshop, and appreciate the efforts of the UNAIDS Asia and Pacific Regional Office, the staff of the IAS and particularly those of Chloe Swift for supporting the *Thinking Politically* initiative. The views are those of the authors and in the case of Buse do not represent the official position of the UN.

Notes

1. On the pressures on French political science to adjust to more American style practices see Billordo (2005).
2. One exception is Dietrich (2007). Available at http://www.carnegiecouncil.org/resources/journal/21_3/essay/001.html/_res/id=sa_File1/Dietrich.pdf.
3. But see Ditmore et al. (2010).
4. The journal *Health & Human Rights* remains testimony to how significant this shift has been. See, for example, Gruskin et al. (2007).

References

Aids2031 Consortium, 2010. *AIDS taking a long-term view*. New Jersey: FT Press.
Allen, T. and Heald, S., 2004. HIV/AIDS policy in Africa: what has worked in Uganda and what has failed in Botswana. *Journal of International Development*, 16 (8), 1141–1154.
Altman, D., 1986. *AIDS in the mind of America*. New York: Doubleday.

Altman, D., 1994. *Power and community*. London: Taylor & Francis.
Altman, D., 2001. *Global sex*. University of Chicago Press.
Altman, D., 2010. Exporting moralities. *In*: P. Aggleton and R. Parker, eds. *Routledge handbook of sexuality, health and rights*. Oxon: Routledge, 37–44.
Andriote, J.-M., 1999. *Victory deferred: how AIDS changed gay life in America*. Chicago: University of Chicago Press.
Berkman, A., et al., 2005. A critical analysis of the Brazilian response to HIV/AIDS: lessons learned for controlling and mitigating the epidemic in developing countries. *American Journal of Public Health*, 95 (7), 1162–1172.
Berridge, V. and Strong, P., eds., 1993. *AIDS and contemporary history*. Cambridge: Cambridge University Press.
Billordo, L., 2005. Publishing in French political science journals: an inventory of methods and sub-fields. *French Politics*, 3 (2), 178–186.
Bor, J., 2007. The political economy of AIDS leadership in developing countries: an exploratory analysis. *Social Science and Medicine*, 64 (8), 1585–1599.
Brown, G. and Labonte, R., 2011. Globalization and its methodological discontents: contextualizing globalization through the study of HIV/AIDS. *Globalization & Health*, 7 (29). Available from: http://www.globalizationandhealth.com/content/7/1/29
Buse, K., et al., 2009. Political feasibility of scaling-up five evidence informed HIV policies: in search of deeper and wider policy commitment. *Sexually Transmitted Infections*, 85 (Suppl. 2), ii37–ii42.
Butler, A., 2005. South Africa's HIV/AIDS policy 1994–2004: how can it be explained? *African Affairs*, 104 (417), 591–614.
Carrillo, H., 2002. *The night is young sexuality in Mexico in the time of AIDS*. Chicago: University Chicago Press.
Crimp, D. ed., 1988. *AIDS: cultural analysis, cultural activism*. Cambridge, MA: MIT Press.
de la Dehesa, R. and Mukherjea, A., 2012. Building capacities and producing citizens: the biopolitics of HIV prevention in Brazil. *Contemporary Politics*, 18 (2), 186–199.
Derman, E., 2011. Unruly humans vs. the lust for order. *New Scientist*, 212 (2835), 32–33.
Dietrich, J.W., 2007. The politics of PEPFAR: the president's emergency plan for AIDS relief. *Ethics and International Affairs*, 21 (3). Available from: http://www.carnegiecouncil.org/resources/journal/21_3/essay/001.html
Ditmore, M.H., Levy, A., and Willman, A., ed., 2010. *Sex work matters: exploring money, power and intimacy in the sex industry*. London: Zed Books.
Dow, U., 2000. *Far and beyond*. Botswana: Longman.
Eberstadt, N., 2002. The future of AIDS. *Foreign Affairs*, 81 (6), 22–45.
England, R., 2008. The writing is on the wall for UNAIDS. *British Medical Journal*, 336, 1072.
England, R., 2011. A strategic revolution in HIV and global health. *The Lancet*, 378 (9787), 226.
Epstein, H., 2007. *The invisible cure: AIDS, the west and the fight against AIDS*. London: Penguin Group.
Epstein, S., 1996. *Impure science: AIDS, activism, and the politics of knowledge*. Berkeley: University of California Press.
Fassin, D., 2007. *When bodies remember: experiences and politics of AIDS in South Africa*. Berkeley: University California Press.
Fillieule, O. and Voegtli, M., 2012. Constitution, diversification and normalization of a health problem: organizing the fight against AIDS in Switzerland (1984–2005). *Contemporary Politics*, 18 (2), 200–212.
Fourie, P. and Follér, M., 2012. AIDS hyper-epidemics and social resilience: theorising the political. *Contemporary Politics*, 18 (2), 254–268.
Frasca, T., 2005. *AIDS in Latin America*. New York: Palgrave.
Friedman, S. and Mottiar, S., 2004. *A moral to the tale: the treatment action campaign and the politics of HIV/AIDS*. Johannesburg: Centre for Policy Studies, University of the Witwatersrand.
Gauri, V. and Lieberman, E.S., 2006. Boundary institutions and HIV/AIDS policy in Brazil and South Africa. *Studies in Comparative International Development*, 41 (3), 47–73.
Geffen, N., 2010. *Debunking delusions*. Cape Town: Jacana Media.
Gould, D., 2009. *Moving politics*. Chicago: Chicago University Press.
Gruskin, S., Mills, E., and Tarantola, D., 2007. History, principles and practice of health and human rights. *The Lancet*, 370, 449–455.
Hawkes, S., et al., 2012. Managing research evidence to inform action: influencing HIV policy to protect marginalised populations in Pakistan. *Global Public Health*, 7 (5), 482–494.

Heald, S., 2006. Abstain or die: the development of HIV/AIDS policy in Botswana. *Journal of Biosocial Science*, 38, 29–41.

Kane, S., 1998. *AIDS alibis: sex, drugs and crime in the Americas*. Philadelphia: Temple University Press.

Kaplan, R., 1997. *The ends of the earth*. London: Papermac.

Kaufman, J., 2012. China's evolving AIDS policy: the influence of global norms and transnational non-governmental organizations. *Contemporary Politics*, 18 (2), 225–238.

Kempadoo, K. and Doezema, J., 1998. *Global sex workers*. London: Routledge.

Kendall, T. and Lopez-Uribe, E., 2010, Improving the HIV response for women in Latin America: barriers to integrated advocacy for sexual and reproductive health and rights. *Global Health Governance*, IV (1). Available from: www.ghgj.org/Kendall%20and%Lopez_final.pdf

Kippax, S. and Holt, M., 2009. *The state of social and political science research related to HIV*. Report for the International AIDS Society, Geneva.

Lasswell, H., 1936. *Politics: who gets what, when, how*. New York: McGraw Hill.

Lieberman, E.S., 2007. Ethnic politics, risk, and policy-making: a cross-national statistical analysis of government responses to HIV/AIDS. *Comparative Political Studies*, 40 (12), 1407.

Lomax Cook, F., *et al.*, 1983. Media and agenda setting: effects on the public, interest group leaders, policy makers, and policy. *Public Opinion Quarterly*, 47 (1), 16–35.

McMichael, A.J., 2009. *Climate change and human health, in commonwealth secretariat, commonwealth health ministers update*. London: Pro-Book, 11–20.

Nutely, S., Walter, I., and Davies, H.T.O., 2007. *Using evidence: how research can inform public services*. Bristol: Policy Press.

O'Keefe, M., 2012. Lessons from the rise and fall of the military AIDS hypothesis: politics, evidence and persuasion. *Contemporary Politics*, 18 (2), 239–253.

Ooms, G., *et al.*, 2008. The diagonal approach to global fund financing. *Globalization and Health*, 4 (6). Available from: http://www.globalizationandhealth.com/content/4/1/6

Parker, R., 2011. Grassroots activism, civil society mobilisation and the politics of the global HIV/AIDS epidemic. *Brown Journal of World Affairs*, xvii (ii), 21–37.

Parkhurst, J. and Lush, L., 2004. The political environment of HIV: lessons from a comparison of Uganda and South Africa. *Social Science & Medicine*, 59 (9), 1913–1924.

Patterson, A. S. & Stephens, D., 2012. AIDS mobilisation in Zambia and Vietnam: explaining the differences. *Contemporary Politics*, 18 (2), 213–224.

Patton, C., 1985. *Sex and germs: the politics of AIDS*. Boston: South End.

Paxton, N.A., 2012. Political science(s) and HIV: a critical analysis. *Contemporary Politics*, 18 (2), 141–155.

Putzel, J., 2004. The politics of action on AIDS: a case study of Uganda. *Public Administration and Development*, 24 (1), 19–30.

Putzel, J., 2006. A history of state action: the politics of AIDS in Uganda and Senegal. *In*: P. Denis and C. Becker, eds. *The HIV/AIDS epidemic in sub-Saharan Africa in a historical perspective*. 171–184.

Sabatier, P., 1988. An advocacy coalition model of policy change and the role of policy-oriented learning therein. *Policy Sciences*, 21 (2–3), 129–168.

Schneider, H., 2002. On the fault-line: the politics of AIDS policy in contemporary South Africa. *African Studies*, 61 (1), 145–167.

Schneider, H. and Stein, J., 2001. Implementing AIDS policy in post-apartheid South Africa. *Social Science and Medicine*, 52, 723–731.

Schwartländer, B., *et al.*, 2011. Towards an improved investment approach for an effective response to HIV/AIDS. *The Lancet*, 377 (9782), 2031–2041.

Sendziuk, P., 2003. *Learning to trust: Australian responses to AIDS*. Sydney: UNSW Press.

Shilts, R., 1987. *And the band played on: politics, people, and the AIDS epidemic*. New York: St Martin's Press.

Smith, J. and Whiteside, A., 2010. The history of AIDS exceptionalism. *Journal of the International AIDS Society*, 13 (1), 47.

Specter, M., 2004. The devastation. *The New Yorker*, 11 October. Available from: http://www.newyorker.com/archive/2004/10/11/041011fa_fact1

Steinberg, J., 2008. *Sizwe's test: a young man's journey through Africa's AIDS epidemic*. New York: Simon & Schuster.

Strand, P., 2012. Public opinion as leadership disincentive: exploring a governance dilemma in the AIDS response in Africa. *Contemporary Politics*, 18 (2), 174–185.

The Economist, 2011. The thinking capital. *The Economist*, 28 April, vol. 57. Available from: http://www.economist.com/node/18618772

United Nations General Assembly, 2001. *United Nations General Assembly Special Session on HIV/AIDS Declaration of Commitment on HIV/AIDS*, 25–27 June. New York: United Nations.

United Nations General Assembly, 2006. *60/262 Political Declaration on HIV/AIDS*. New York: United Nations.

United Nations General Assembly, 2011. *Political Declaration on HIV/AIDS: Intensifying Our Efforts to Eliminate HIV/AIDS*, 7 June. New York: United Nations.

United Nations Security Council, 2000. *UN Security Council Resolution 1308 on the Responsibility of the Security Council in the Maintenance of International Peace and Security: HIV/AIDS and International Peace-Keeping Operations*. New York: United Nations.

de Waal, A., 2003. Human rights organisations and the political imagination: how the west and Africa have diverged. *Journal of Human Rights*, 2 (4), 475–494.

de Waal, A. Klot, J.F., and Mahajan, M., 2010. *HIV/AIDS, security and conflict*. New York: Social Science Research Council.

Ward, V., House, A., and Hamer, S., 2009. Developing a framework for transferring knowledge into action: a thematic analysis of the literature. *Journal of Health Services Research and Policy*, 14 (3), 156–164.

Watney, S., 1986. *Policing desire: pornography, AIDS and the media*. London: Comedia.

Political science(s) and HIV: a critical analysis

Nathan A. Paxton

The academic discipline of political science has substantially addressed the politics and policy of the HIV/AIDS epidemic over the last two decades, but the epidemic has not become a full-fledged research agenda of its own. The author analyses and groups the extant research into four research programmes. He suggests some future directions that political science may take, so as to further the investigation of the empirical problem of HIV/AIDS, as well as to meet the disciplinary imperative to advance more general theories and explanations of political phenomena.

Introduction

In the 30 years that we have recognised HIV's existence among us, we have encountered a disease requiring and entailing an engagement like no other of academic scientists with policy-makers, activists, and politicians. This epidemic, perhaps more than any other recent communicable disease or naturally derived phenomenon, has required the collaboration of social and natural sciences to find viable solutions to the problem of its spread.

The political aspects of the epidemic cannot be ignored, nor can they be left to natural scientists or politicians. The world has need for the expertise of politics scholars in the same way it needs that of economists. At their best, these scholars can stand apart from short-term or partisan views, to point out alternatives, analogues, and paths not taken in this issue area or in parallel ones. Political sciences have the potential to make a unique contribution to the study of and response to the epidemic, oriented as they are to the explanation of decision-making actors, institutions, ideas, and processes. Political science has produced a large amount of research into the epidemic, but it has occurred across a wide variety of research programmes and traditions. This article discusses the several ways that the political sciences have addressed the worldwide epidemic, with an eye towards taking a categorical and critical view of the supply of academic political research. I discuss four research programmes into which political scientists have ensconced research on HIV, noting strengths and weaknesses and assessing the extent of coverage and elisions.

I attempt to take a fairly catholic view of what constitutes 'political science' in this analysis. A full discussion is beyond the scope or focus of this article, but in broad terms the major divide as to what constitutes a political science falls along the lines of disciplinarity and geography. North Americans tend to see themselves as members of a coherent discipline of 'political science' with its own departments, associations, values, criteria for research acceptability, and differentiation from other academic fields. In the rest of the world, social scientists who study politics work more interdisciplinarily and accept a greater range of epistemology and methodologies as legitimate fur use in research.

Scholars using HIV as a substantive focus have contributed to a broad range of theoretical research programmes, across the range of the discipline. That said, there has been and remains the impression that political science is uninterested in the epidemic.

The number of works that address the politics of the epidemic in a social scientific fashion and in a form recognisable to academic practitioners as constituting 'political science' is substantial. In larger terms, however, it does not constitute a coherent research programme of its own, and it has constituted a substantial portion of only one or two research programmes.

Political science has considered four major aspects of the HIV epidemic, integrating those into its concerns with the political world.

(1) the growth and extension of global and comparative health policy;
(2) how the spread of the epidemic has affected the progress of international development;
(3) effects on state security environments, internally and externally;
(4) how HIV's politics have affected and been affected by trends in governance, on all political levels.

Once separated into these substantive research agendas, we see many of the same approaches and types of questions recurring across agendas. Institutional analysis, administrative quality and changes, and the emergence and environment of civil society recur often. The research question generally involves delineating the relations among affected actors, as well as examining the use of power and politics in those relations. Some research begins from relatively theoretical questions, and investigation leads to better understanding of the results of public policy decisions and regimes. Other research starts from public policy concerns, and it ties into theoretical and scientific agendas.

Global and comparative health

Over the last 15 years, political researchers have turned their attention to the socio-political problems of health and disease that inhere in a globalised society. The system of identifying and managing disease outbreaks has necessarily exceeded the grasp of any one country, no matter how powerful it is in conventional terms.

Human health is a good that relies upon the coordination and cooperation of a variety of global, national, and international actors in a variety of frameworks, institutions, and organisations. Political researchers have examined the formation and functioning of global institutions to manage the spread of HIV; the provision of resources for treatment and prevention; and the establishment of scientific, governmental, and activist bodies and networks of cooperation. Some global health politics research also examines the institutional relations and inter-/intra-organisational politics of these actors, while other research has sought to understand what policies have come from the health regime's actors. Social movements research has attempted to understand how activists use the instruments at their disposal to expand health regimes and policies.

State performance

One of the most significant questions that politics scholars have engaged with respect to global and comparative health has been in understanding how differences in societies affect the scope and intensity of anti-HIV response.

Cultural explanatory models have proved popular and persuasive. The different policy regimes that various African states undertook, based on political culture – 'the dynamic and heterogeneous ground of collective identities, ideologies, and historical pathways of different political forces' – explain a large part of the differing paths Cameroon, Côte d'Ivoire, Senegal, South Africa, and Uganda took (Eboko 2005, p. 38). Patriarchy underlies many of the features of African governance (Siplon 2005). With women excluded from many of the highest levels of power, there are fewer advocates for strong national HIV responses, along with a number of policy choke-points that can render even the best intentioned and resourced programmes ineffectual. Altman (2006) focuses upon sexual culture and mores; these taboos surrounding uncomfortable topics go a long way towards explaining why governments fail to implement policies and programmes, even when the outcomes are clear and beneficial.

Another strand of policy output research contends that the main causal factors explaining differential state action are organisational or institutional in nature. Comparing Uganda and South Africa in the 1990s, Parkhurst and Lush (2004) focused on four aspects of political institutions: political leadership; extant bureaucracies and configuration; health systems and infrastructure; and what governments allow or assign non-governmental organisations (NGOs) and civil society organisations (CSOs) to do. As they point out, government organisation and bureaucratic performance appear to have a strong effect upon a country's policy output performance. Allen and Heald (2004), comparing Botswana and Uganda, argued that leaders' engagement helped ameliorate the problems occurring with 'one-size-fits-all' prevention strategies. A country's degree of press freedom, income equality, and overall HIV prevalence can explain much of political leaders' commitment (Bor 2007). Culture and institutions can mutually reinforce each other. Lieberman investigates the independent variable of 'boundary institutions': the 'sets of rules that regulate racial and ethnic group categories and intergroup behaviour' (Gauri and Lieberman 2006, p. 46). Although 'boundary institutions' are not identical to sub-national or ethnic identities, boundary institutions depend upon cultural identity constructs. Removing the institutions may therefore not change policy output, due to the underlying cultural constraints. Boundary institutions that reinforce cultural identities can impede the design, implementation, and output of anti-HIV policies, due to different degrees of risk perception for in- and out-group members (Lieberman 2009).

Some studies investigate a 'tough case' version of the question above ('why are some countries better performers than others?'). Elbe (2002) explained how a poor country with recent civil strife and little democracy (Uganda) was able to get in front of the epidemic. As President Museveni became aware of the extent of HIV infection in the military, he worked to curtail the disease, because the military was his power base and provided general social stability. Youde (2005) traced South Africa's failure to implement a treatment programme to a 'fundamental disjuncture' between South African politicians and the international HIV epistemic community, giving rise to a counter-community in South Africa.

States in partnership for health

States have not managed to build policy solutions that work without coordinated action among various types of actors, either under their own auspices or by delegation to other entities. For researchers interested in how states interact with actors like NGOs and multi-national corporations (MNCs), study of the global and comparative health regimes has provided a number of examples.

The requisite role of states or other actor types is yet indeterminate. While states rely upon and partner with non-state actors under the best of circumstances, in a number of countries, NGOs and corporations have addressed the pandemic when the state government has failed to do much. NGOs are seen at the 'forefront' of the response, with influence over government and international organisation (IO) activity (Clarke 2002), and the state and its structures sometimes do not figure very much in fighting the pandemic (Barnes 2008). Others point out that cooperative efforts between state and civil society, or the development of 'policy networks', are crucial for policy agenda-setting, development, and implementation (Tantivess and Walt 2008). In other research, central or national governments are necessary; research on Uganda and Senegal indicates that an effective and sufficient response requires central government involvement (Putzel 2006). Sometimes the interaction between states and their non-governmental partners is formalised in a 'public–private partnership' (PPP) (Ramiah and Reich 2006). The organisational aspect of these partnerships – particularly institutional memory and stability – cannot be neglected, given the potentially high rates of attrition for local staff who are HIV-positive or care for someone who is (James and Mullins 2004).

Why does collaboration between state and non-state actors either fail to coalesce or break down? Such collaboration apparently depends upon the civil society environment generally. In Ghana, a unique case of a state that transitioned to democracy and where HIV seemed to be at a critical point between control and crisis, a broad response to HIV has not developed, due at least in part to a relatively weak civil society (Haven and Patterson 2007). South Africa's difficulties in the period when both HIV and AIDS were on the rise (particularly the 1990s) were legion, involving the 'difficulties of implementing a comprehensive response to AIDS in a country undergoing restructuring at every level' (Schneider and Stein 2001, p. 723).

Corporations face consequences from the pandemic, and relations with the state can hinder or help companies' actions against HIV. South African corporations were slow to address HIV, given the potential economic losses from employee morbidity and mortality (Dickinson 2004). Corporations face complex socio-economic cleavages or race, class, gender, and their confluences, and the companies lack the power to resolve them. In the southern African mining sector, companies in reality have little financial incentive to prevent employee infection, miners' unions lack institutional power, and government ministries are subject to capture and lack bureaucratic capacity (Stuckler *et al*. 2010, pp. 5–7). The regional nature of mining makes it hard for any one state to address.

International and global governmental organisations have also played important roles in the political management of HIV. HIV responses demonstrate both the workings of international institutions and the changing basis of relations between citizens and the state, at least *vis-à-vis* supranational institutions. One of the most important shifts has been in the role that IOs, NGOs, and CSOs have played in the formation and work of organisations like WHO's Global Programme on AIDS; its successor, UNAIDS; the Global Fund; and so forth (Gómez 2009). NGOs have also played a role in the formation and implementation of policies and norms, with the support of and independent of national government support (Swidler 2006).

The HIV pandemic has provided some researchers with an excellent opportunity to examine what happens when global institutions and local programmes partner directly. There can be a disjuncture between the international institutions of global response that set the priorities for policy, expenditure, and prioritisation and the localised realities that shape people's experience and understanding of the disease; global actors often do not see how their efforts play out both in limited space and medium-term time (Seckinelgin 2008). Local actors in Kenya, Malawi, and Zambia sensed a lack of coordination among different global donor programmes. Consultative mechanisms that bring local concerns and ideas to global implements and funders have, for example, improved treatment and care of people living with HIV and AIDS (PLWHA), as well as improve acceptance and adherence to care programmes (Edström and MacGregor 2010, Mallouris *et al*. 2010).

Social movements and activism

Social movements, identity politics, and activism enjoy an active and well-consolidated research agenda in political science. From the beginning, identity politics has played one of the most important roles in the formation of the movements around HIV. In part, this is because HIV first manifested in the developed/northern countries in gay men; it drew upon, merged with, and provided fuel for the lesbian and gay rights movements that had begun one to two decades previous. Scholarship on gay and lesbian activism in the last 30 years has thus had to grapple with the place of the HIV pandemic in the movement. Gay men (and to lesser degrees, lesbians, haemophiliacs, and those who worked with injecting drug users and immigrants) pressured governments, rich community members, medical professionals, and others to step up research and care, speed drug approval, provide legal protections against discrimination, cooperate in medical decision-making, and include PLWHA in decision-making (Smith and Siplon 2006).

Outside of the USA, gay liberation and HIV activism co-occurred regularly. In Mexico and Brazil, the emergence of HIV among men who have sex with men provided a spur to sexual minorities to organise around their political and civil rights (de la Dehesa 2010). Sex workers in Southeast Asia and Latin America have often used their marginal social status and 'otherness' to create, refine, or re-invigorate strong collective identity and to make demands for protections and changes. In Singapore and Malaysia, the HIV movement 'allowed them to play critical roles in spurring and supporting queer – especially GLBT [gay, lesbian, bisexual, transgender] – mobilisation, including fostering a sense of a "gay community", despite legal proscriptions on homosexual behaviour and associations' (Weiss 2006, p. 674).

In sub-Saharan Africa, identity politics has relied upon a person's HIV status itself to be the marker of identity. Some studies point to the difficulty of organising around identity, as HIV-positive status alone may not be sufficient to create an activist movement. In Tanzania, HIV activism has not (yet) had very much of a political impact, in part for this reason of identity basis (Beckmann and Bujra 2010). In Ghana, newly consolidated democracy, weak civil society, and a very small or marginal identity politics lobby has resulted in little political attention or action on HIV (Patterson 2006).

South Africa has demonstrated a particularly robust activist movement. In particular, the success of the treatment action campaign (TAC) has provoked analysis on alternatives to identity politics. TAC – along with its partner, MSF (Medecins Sans Frontieres) – avoided conflict over the origins of HIV. Instead it devoted itself to 'class-based politics that concentrated on access to anti-retroviral drugs' (Robins 2004). Heywood (2009), on the other hand, contends that the TAC focused on human rights discourse over other sources of political coherence and power.

Identity can also have pernicious effects, especially when different identities cut against one another. Youde (2005, 2007) found that South African political elites' self-identity of independence and anti-colonialism, combined with the legacies of apartheid, formed an 'epistemic community' that culminated in Mbeki's denialism. For African-Americans, where identity politics cut against acknowledging and addressing HIV, PLWHA experienced 'secondary marginalisation' (Cohen 1999).

International development

HIV has not been spread equally around the world. Countries in lower and middle income tiers have borne the greatest burden of this disease, with sub-Saharan Africa particularly hard-hit. These are also countries that have been engaged in continuing programmes of socio-economic development. Two questions about the relationship of HIV to development have tended to dominate. The first has been to examine how the pandemic has affected development gains made in the last 50–75 years. The other dominant question asks how the international community has changed its ideas about development assistance in light of the widespread, slow-moving epidemic disaster that HIV has proved to be. Unlike many other communicable epidemic diseases, HIV appears slowly, proves biologically challenging to fight, and appears to spread best under political conditions of discrimination, stigmatisation, and human rights violations. These conditions add to the complexities of a challenging endeavour.

It is largely uncontroversial that HIV threatens development in the countries of sub-Saharan Africa. The changes that donor and partner governments and organisations have asked of African countries and peoples – such as rapid changes in gender roles, Western understandings of sexuality and sexual behaviour, the denial of denial, and so forth – may be necessary from a biomedical or epidemiological perspective, but they also engender many African countries' perceptions of re-colonisation (Fredland 1998). The tragedy of South African policy under Thabo Mbeki has at least part of its basis in this cause (Schneider 2002, Butler 2005).

In the late 1990s and early 2000s, a near-universal condition for debt reduction and write-down was 'structural readjustment'. Although structural readjustment may have freed monies to do such things as fight HIV, the reduction of the state's role in the economy and society mean that it may not have the reach to tackle HIV comprehensively or effectively (Poku 2002, Whiteside 2002).

Indeed, the policies required for structural adjustment programmes created conditions that spread HIV more effectively (Poku and Sandkjaer 2007, pp. 134–136). Whiteside warned, in this context, that researchers and policymakers have ignored HIV too much in development policies, forgetting that HIV is a long-wave, inter-generational event, where the effects will play out for decades, even if the disease itself were to stop tomorrow (Whiteside 2006).

Politics has proved a vital ingredient in the success the HIV response has enjoyed in developing countries. Political activity, issue framing, and strategic communication may be equally or more central to raising and furthering particular global health issues like HIV than demonstrating the burden of a particular disease or the cost-effectiveness of treatment. The policy community around HIV has better advanced its ideas regarding problems and solutions, and they have better institutionalised these ideas, which in turn increases the attention the policy community can gain from policymakers (Shiffman 2009).

Much of the rich world's response to HIV in the developing world has relied in great measure upon the work of various types of NGOs: medical, political, advocacy, humanitarian, and religious. The proliferation of these organisations makes them virtually indispensable to the fight against HIV (Clarke 2002, White and Morton 2005). International donors and funders often seem to prefer NGOs to government involvement, both because NGOs are perceived to be more free-form or 'local' (and thus potentially more flexible and responsive) and because there can be concerns about the ability or corruption of governments. It often seems the developed world considers Africans too poor, too unsophisticated, too corrupt, or too sexual to adequately handle treatment programmes (Jones 2004).

Worries exist, however, that NGOs reproduce or create new forms of colonialism. Locals, 'at least initially, inevitably regard an international organisation as a potential source of money, goods or contacts that are otherwise unavailable' (Swidler 2006, p. 277). As time passes, there is often a mismatch, culturally and politically, between the NGOs' ways of doing and those of the encompassing society.

HIV assistance policies meant to be sustainable serve to highlight extant power inequalities while creating new ones. In Malawi, HIV assistance has exacerbated the problems of a class of 'interstitial elites'. These elites – who mediate between national and foreign NGO staff in the national capital and local village chiefs or heads – are relatively capable and educated but expected to volunteer their efforts. These interstitial elites exist in fiscal, social and professional insecurity and they are more and more dependent upon irregular payments (Swidler and Watkins 2009).

HIV has also provided developing countries with the means by which they can and have resisted the preferences of developed countries and pursue their own preferences, through institutions above and alongside developing countries.

States and IOs are hardly powerless in the face of MNCs. Research into drug manufacturers' decision to begin producing generic anti-retroviral therapies (ARVs) in 2001 shows that governments created markets for generics by altering regulatory environments and 'buying drugs for people living with HIV in developing countries' (Roemer-Mahle 2010, p. 9), and countries have been able to leverage international intellectual property (IP) law regimes against drug manufacturers and their home countries (Cleary and Ross 2002, Cullet 2003). IP rights regimes create a scarcity in knowledge, increasing their economic value but which also increases dependence on the state. Rights-holders, like pharma companies, cannot let the costs of their goods become too high, lest the state cease rights enforcement (May 2007).

The most well known of these IP law resistance actions took place with respect to the TRIPs (trade-related aspects of IP rights) agreement and the Doha round of the World Trade Organization talks. The TRIPs agreement, although often interpreted as being to the benefit of developed countries and 'big pharma', contains provisions that were leveraged against the same. Developing countries have used the tools of 'national emergency', and 'compulsory licenses' to local manufacturers to extract more favourable terms, under threat of depriving the pharmaceutical producers of further revenues (Sell 2007). Furthermore, developing countries re-framed the access problem, such that appeals to norms, ethics, and legitimacy became the terms of the debate over generic ARVs. Powerful actors were internationally shamed, and the eventual result was the 2001 Doha Declaration on the TRIPs Agreement and Public Health. This opens new possibilities of action in international politics, especially for South-South cooperation. These cooperative engagements can allow for creative and perfectly legal ways around TRIPs and Doha (Aginam 2010).

Country-specific analyses have helped to illuminate how developing nations have sometimes defied of current trends or the wishes of the powerful in international development. Brazil has proved particularly interesting for analysis because it sits at the intersection of 'local, foreign, and transnational actors. ... The full mobilisation of Brazil's government, both in its relations with the USA and in international forums, as well as the support this government received from transnational advocacy networks were critical in enabling it to resist ... pressures' from developed country governments and major pharmaceutical companies (de Mello e Souza 2007, pp. 37–38).

Security

One of the primary foci of international relations is the concern with how a polity protects itself internally and with respect to other polities. The traditional focus of such inquiry has been upon interstate war, but with the end of the Cold War, studies of civil and ethnic warfare became more prominent. Expansion of what 'security' encompassed also arose, as 'human security' – which looks to the factors that make human beings, not just states, safer – took greater prominence. Significant analysis has focused on how HIV may pose either a traditional or human security threat.

Elbe (2006) cautions against tying HIV too tightly into the security paradigm, for 'securitisation' of the disease has implications beyond simply raising its priority on a country's preference agenda. Securitisation could allow for more space to move a country's response from civilian control to military control, thereby affecting civil liberties and the balance of power between military and civilian leaders. Militarising or securitising HIV also creates a greater possibility that care for elites and military heads will be formally prioritised, and it mitigates against continued efforts at normalisation of the disease.

Several questions have emerged linking HIV and security. There is the question of whether HIV constitutes a threat in traditional or in human security terms. There are also studies that examine how HIV might affect the (generally traditional) security position and posture of states. Finally, there are studies that investigate how war and conflict affect or exacerbate the problem of HIV in developing societies.

The causal pathway linking HIV to security is a difficult one to trace (Barnett 2006). HIV sunders fundamental social units, like the linkage of grandparent to parent to child, as it kills off parents and leaves the elderly to raise the young. Although analysts can explain that such change in fundamental institutions will 'hollow out civil society', the exact repercussions are unclear and HIV is a (large) part of a complex of factors and causes breaking down trust between government and citizens (Price-Smith 2002). Traditional security studies scholars have hewed close to examining HIV as the cause or consequence of war and peace, violent conflict, and state survival (for an overview of a recent comprehensive research programme, see de Waal 2010b). Some connections between HIV and state security are sensible and substantiated. States with a norm of international cooperation are more likely to identify HIV as a security threat, and states seeking foreign investment are more likely to de-emphasise the HIV-security linkage (Girshick 2004). HIV does not seem to pose a threat to the security postures of the rich, developed countries like the USA; in poorer countries, it has a high degree of association with human rights abuses and civil conflict (Peterson 2003).

In other cases, the connections are harder to piece together. Examining the Security Council's claims in 2000 that HIV posed risks to state stability, national security, peacekeeping operations, and that violence exacerbates the virus's spread, McInnes (2006) noted that the evidence since 2000 showed the linkages to be less clear, more complex, and more case-dependent. HIV is a long-term event – the dying-off of the infected is only the first effect the disease will have on populations (Barnett 2006). There is perhaps 20 years of evidence available, providing only the most basic understanding of what will happen to these complex systems, and so short-term actions may be as damaging as helpful to the long-term situation.

The relationship of HIV and the conduct of war is complex and indeterminate in both causal directions. On a micro-level, Elbe (2002) noted that HIV has become one of the weapons that armed groups deploy; rape of civilian populations becomes more terrifying a tactic when rolled up with the peril of infection. Experience and anecdotes from IO, NGO, and other observers solidified a consensus around how war and sexual violence spread HIV. However, controversial work (Spiegel 2004, Spiegel *et al.* 2007) examined the epidemiology of HIV prevalence in the presence of conflict; no consistent relationship could be found. To the contrary, Iqbal and Zorn (2010) find a 'clear, positive relationship' between war and increased prevalence of HIV, indicating that wars do affect the progress of the epidemic. Some work considers the effect that HIV may have on military structure and organisations. Rosen (1987), for example, provided early theorising that HIV could damage military efficacy. Since prevalence is often higher in the military than in the general population, we should expect to see a greater proportion of the military's personnel contracting HIV; this decreases the activity of those individuals (with their skills and experience) from the organisation. This can eventually lead to decreased organisational effectiveness and increased instability.

Most empirical confirmation of such arguments have taken place in the sub-Saharan African context. Ostergard (2002) discusses the effects of HIV upon the military in a number of countries, with attention to Nigeria, DR Congo, and Uganda. Elbe (2002) notes that African militaries have experienced loss of organisational capacity and lowered effectiveness, using descriptive statistics from several countries. Within sub-Saharan Africa, because many militaries engage in extended peacekeeping missions, higher levels of HIV in the ranks will affect peacekeeping abilities and operations in the region (Patel and Tripodi 2007).

High prevalence of HIV in the military has increased the incidence of illness and death. While militaries are designed to address the problem of large-scale personnel loss, challenges remain. HIV pushes militaries functionally and organisational as they grow beyond conventional competencies: dealing with post-conflict situations, getting civilians and military leaders to learn from one another in their HIV control strategies, and increasing the HIV readiness and response of paramilitary organisations (de Waal 2010a). Soldiers cannot carry out their duties at an increasing rate, and this affects staffing decisions, as well as recruitment and conscription needs.

Governance

The governance of a society – the interrelation of government, economy, civil society, citizens, and private enterprise to *one another* and how those joint interactions shape and constrain 'public affairs' – is a major concern for political scientists. Those who study governance 'explore abstract analyses of the construction of social orders, social coordination, or social practices irrespective of their specific content' (Bevir 2007, p. 365). A particular concern of this research agenda has been in examining how various public sector reforms to lessen the hierarchy and centralisation of social functions in government. HIV experienced a coincident rise with such trends in public sector management, and many attempts to address the pandemic have relied upon a variety of non-state actors, including NGOs, private enterprises, PPPs, and special-purpose global organisations, among others.

To some degree, the governance research agenda overlaps with elements of the preceding research programmes. It differs in that rather than focus on the particular *issues* of content, governance studies examine the question of *how or how should* a society self-manage, the *justifications*, and the *ends* of such management. Here HIV is interesting not only for its own political implications, nor as a sub-topic of a larger class of political phenomena, but because of what it tells us of the interior and exterior understanding of the society.

Several pertinent questions arise:

- What effects does the disease have on the state and society? How does HIV change the social and political institutions of the state?
- Why do some states fail so utterly in responding and even well-managed states 'miss' the problem of HIV? How does the epidemic bring the state's pathologies into focus?
- How do countries' HIV responses demonstrate the well-functioning of the state and its components?

The first question ponders how the effects upon aggregated individuals bring demographic, political, economic, and other social impacts into being.

> ... [T]he pandemic threatens structural transformations in African economies, institutions and governance. Decreased adult life expectancy has important adverse impacts upon savings, capital accumulation, skills acquisition, and institutional functioning. ... [T]he impacts of the pandemic can be envisaged as running processes of demographic transition, economic development and the growth of a bureaucratic state, in reverse. (de Waal 2003, p. 12)

HIV affects social function and stability in sub-Saharan Africa because it can radically deplete human capital. It strains medical facilities already under pressure, increases the risk of infection due to the disruptions caused by refugee flows, pushes HIV into rural areas via urbanisation or civil conflict, and 'inverts priorities' (Elbe 2002) for all sorts of people, as day-to-day survival becomes more pressing than infection avoidance. de Waal (2010a) notes that militaries have often been faster and more effective than other parts of their governments to deal with the human capital costs of HIV. Some institutions and organisations, however, will suffer an inversion of priorities, as workers take time off or quit outright to care for themselves or family members; and as human, economic, and political capital must be expended upon HIV prevention, control, and treatment rather than other facets of social development.

HIV response management signals the politico-technical capacity of a government and society to national and international publics; it is a sign of governmental competence and legitimacy (Compton 2007). Especially when setting up programmes, there is often a failure to appreciate that HIV is a problem of governance: many actors seek remedy in 'an organisational fix' rather than facing the 'political challenge of prioritising HIV/AIDS in government and non-government sectors' (Putzel 2004a, p. 1137).However, at least with respect to the Global Fund, adaptation over time has led to more efficient use of resources as countries have better fit required national-level structures into local context (Dickinson and Druce 2010).

On a philosophical level, the nexus of international institution, national government, and NGO bears a particularly North Atlantic mark of 'governmentality': '... the conventional focus on organisational form and getting management technologies right in order to be able to participate in the international policy environment neutralises our understanding of what these NGOs can actually do' (Seckinelgin 2008, p. 69). That is, by co-opting local organisations and institutions, whatever form they originally take, global actors diminish local capacities to have an effect in their environments.

The (mis)management of HIV responses, which is the heart of the second question above, provides opportunity to examine how organisational or leadership pathologies can lead to an active avoidance of the problem, even as evidence mounts that the government's active denial or neglect of that problem contributes to the problem. Well-run countries, whether developed or developing, have demonstrated similar inabilities to recognise the severity of the epidemic. To be effective, HIV management has to rank high on a society's priorities. Where it is not, even capacious, well-run countries can be caught off guard and encounter difficulty catching up to the disease. For example, in the early 1980s, France could have responded forcefully and effectively, but because of emphasis on fiscal austerity, public service privatisation, and the association of the disease with American gays, the French government did not implement prevalence minimisation programmes (Bosia 2006).

Governance in a democracy may not provide the 'right' incentives for leaders to address the pandemic because HIV requires a more sustained, long-term point of view. Strand (2010) points out a contradiction at the heart of what he calls 'democratic AIDS governance': if political leaders show leadership on HIV, especially in East and Southern African contexts, they encounter opposing populist politics that scapegoat PLWHA and add to discrimination and denial. Democracies may also be short-sighted, with leaders focused only on the next election, but the evidence here is mixed. Dionne (2011) finds that lengthened time horizons are associated with greater funding for HIV, but that shorter time horizons for leaders leads to 'more comprehensive AIDS policy'. One reason HIV has not become an issue in Ghana (which is democratic and well-governed) has been because there has been little to no constituency calling upon political leaders to act (Haven and Patterson 2007).

Democracy may require trade-offs that run counter to maximising anti-HIV policy. One reason for Uganda's relative success under Museveni may have been the regime's lack of democracy. 'The centralist character of the Museveni regime was crucial not only to mobilising state organisations and foreign aid resources, but also to ensuring significant involvement from non-state associations and religious authorities' (Putzel 2004b). Disease emergencies require centralised coordination and distributed instruments for efficient information movement, and these are in tension with one another. Putzel concludes democracy would not have helped

Uganda's response, because the centralist state 'was crucial not only to mobilising state organisations and foreign aid resources, but also to ensuring significant involvement from non-state actors' (p. 29).

The same factors that impede effective state response may also be those that in a different context facilitate action and demonstrate a state's capacity for functioning well. Democracies, for example, may also contain unique institutional advantages that may assist the fight against HIV. The TAC has used constitutional guarantees of human rights, due process of law, and peaceful protest and political pressure to either ally with or defy South Africa's government (Friedman and Mottiar 2004). The tension between hierarchy and distribution exists not only in the state's character but also in its bureaucracy. State organisational configuration matters. Paxton (2010), in qualitative analysis of Mexico and Botswana, finds that when state organs have a networked organisational configuration, they have higher policy responses than those organised as hierarchies or market-anarchies.

Many have attempted to understand the Mbeki regime's vehement biomedical, social, and demographic denialism. Mbeki, however, was only the most extreme example of the trend; a more general denial also occurred in the apartheid, de Klerk, and Mandela administrations. Pursuit of a 'national agenda' of apartheid, nation-building and reconciliation, economic development, or an 'African Renaissance' justified the subversion of all other concerns. HIV served as a political tool for governments to use or ignore, depending on how it integrated with the administration agenda (Fourie and Meyer 2010). South African governments, although inclusive in policy formation post-apartheid, have proved exclusive in (HIV) policy implementation and management. 'Time and again, the South African government acts on a proclivity to want to monopolise such implementation, and when this fails, it reverts to blaming extra-governmental forces. Instead of allowing the explicit bottom-up implementation of these appropriate policy documents, the government has insisted on a top-down approach' (Fourie 2006, p. 179). The effects have been substantial: South Africa has suffered economically, demographically, politically, and as a regional security hegemon. 'The long- and short-term political and economic stability of the entire southern African region will be jeopardised as South Africa becomes less capable of coping with the fallout of the epidemic' (Price-Smith *et al.* 2007, p. 242).

Conclusion

Little more than a decade ago, in a survey of what political science could contribute to addressing the greatest disease epidemic of our time, one article noted, 'Nearly two decades into a pandemic that poses one of the gravest threats to public health and development that sub-Saharan Africa has ever faced, political science can no longer afford to ignore the political implications of AIDS in Africa. A rich array of research agendas linking AIDS and politics is worthy of systematic attention...' (Boone and Batsell 2001, p. 26).

This is not the case on the eve of the first International AIDS Conference to be held in the USA in over 20 years. Political sciences have contributed a grand array and scope of studies, expanding our knowledge and understanding of the socio-political aspects and consequences of this latter-day scourge. The large majority of the research surveyed here has taken place since 2001. This research may not always have fit into a coherent policy agenda, nor has it necessarily moved in directions that policy professionals might prefer. But we know exponentially more now than we did 10 years ago. Plenty of potential research remains, and the possibilities touch on all corners of the systematic study of politics, whether one is interested in responses to HIV *per se* or as an example of some other political phenomenon.

There is much that we still do not know about the interrelationship of this disease with the politics of developed and developing countries. The political sciences, however, are uniquely equipped among disciplines of knowledge to examine how ideas, interests, and institutions relate to power, decisions, and the disease. That, indeed, is the comparative advantage of political science *vis-à-vis* the other social sciences. Political science researchers may not ask or answer exactly the questions that policymakers have. But while in pursuit of advancing the frontiers of knowledge, political researchers can provide foundations for the betterment of the human world.

Acknowledgement

This research was supported by UNAIDS but does not necessarily reflect the policy of UNAIDS.

References

Aginam, O., 2010. Global health governance, intellectual property and access to essential medicines: opportunities and impediments for south-south cooperation. *Global Health Governance*, January. Available from: http://www.ghgj.org/Aginam_final.pdf [accessed 15 April 2010].
Allen, T. and Heald, S., 2004. HIV/AIDS policy in africa: what has worked in uganda and what has failed in botswana? *Journal of International Development*, 16 (8), 1141–1154.
Altman, D., 2006. Taboos and denial in government responses. *International Affairs*, 82 (2), 257–268.
Barnes, N., 2008. Paradoxes and asymmetries of transnational networks: a comparative case study of Mexico's community-based AIDS organizations. *Social Science & Medicine*, 66 (4), 933–944.
Barnett, T., 2006. A long-wave event. HIV/AIDS, politics, governance and 'security': sundering the inter-generational bond? *International Affairs*, 82 (2), 297–313.
Beckmann, N. and Bujra, J., 2010. The 'politics of the queue': the politicization of people living with HIV/AIDS in tanzania. *Development and Change*, 41 (6), 1041–1064.
Bevir, M., 2007. Governance. *Encyclopedia of governance*, vol. 1. Thousand Oaks, CA: Sage Reference, 364–381.
Boone, C. and Batsell, J., 2001. Politics and AIDS in Africa. *Africa Today*, 48 (2), 3–33.
Bor, J., 2007. The political economy of AIDS leadership in developing countries: an exploratory analysis. *Social Science & Medicine*, 64 (8), 1585–1599.
Bosia, M., 2006. Written in blood: AIDS prevention and the politics of failure in France. *Perspectives on Politics*, 4 (4), 647–653.
Butler, A., 2005. South Africa's HIV/AIDS policy, 1994–2004: how can it be explained? *African Affairs*, 104 (417), 591–614.
Clarke, M., 2002. Achieving behaviour change: three generations of HIV/AIDS programming and jargon in Thailand. *Development in Practice*, 12 (5), 625–636.
Cleary, S. and Ross, D., 2002. The 1998–2001 legal struggle between the South African government and the international pharmaceutical industry: a game-theoretic analysis. *Journal of Social, Political and Economic Studies*, 27 (4), 445–494.
Cohen, C.J., 1999. *The boundaries of blackness: AIDS and the breakdown of black politics*. Chicago: University of Chicago Press.
Compton, R., 2007. Dynamics of HIV/AIDS in China and India: assessing government response. *In*: R.L. Ostergard, ed. *HIV/AIDS and the threat to national and international security*. Global Issues Series. Houndmills: Palgrave Macmillan, 223–240.
Cullet, P., 2003. Patents and medicines: the relationship between TRIPs and the human right to health. *International Affairs*, 79 (1), 139–160.
de la Dehesa, R., 2010. *Queering the public sphere in Mexico and Brazil: sexual rights movements in emerging democracies*. Durham: Duke University Press.
Dickinson, C. and Druce, N., 2010. Perspectives integrating country coordinating mechanisms with existing national health and AIDS structures: emerging issues and future directions. *Global Health Governance*, IV (1). Available from: http://blogs.shu.edu/ghg/files/2011/11/Dickinson-and-Druce_Perspectives-Integrating-Country-Coordinating-Mechanisms_Fall-20101.pdf [accessed 15 April 2010].
Dickinson, D., 2004. Corporate South Africa's response to HIV/AIDS: why so slow? *Journal of Southern African Studies*, 30 (3), 627–649.
Dionne, K.Y., 2011. The role of executive time horizons in state response to AIDS in Africa. *Comparative Political Studies*, 44 (1), 55–77.

Eboko, F., 2005. Patterns of mobilization: political culture in the fight against AIDS. *In:* A.S. Patterson, ed. *The African state and the AIDS crisis*. Aldershot: Ashgate, 37–58.

Edström, J. and MacGregor, H., 2010. The pipers call the tunes in global aid for AIDS: the global financial architecture for hiv funding as seen by local stakeholders in Kenya, Malawi and Zambia. *Global Health Governance*, IV (1), 1–12.

Elbe, S., 2002. HIV/AIDS and the changing landscape of war in Africa. *International Security*, 27 (2), 159–177.

Elbe, S., 2006. Should HIV/AIDS be securitized? The ethical dilemmas of linking HIV/AIDS and security. *International Studies Quarterly*, 50 (1), 119–144.

Fourie, P., 2006. *The political management of HIV and AIDS in South Africa: one burden too many?* Basingstoke: Palgrave Macmillan.

Fourie, P. and Meyer, M., 2010. *The politics of AIDS denialism: South Africa's failure to respond*. Global Health. Farnham: Ashgate.

Fredland, R., 1998. AIDS and development: an inverse correlation? *The Journal of Modern African Studies*, 36 (4), 547–568.

Friedman, S. and Mottiar, S., 2004. *Rewarding engagement?: the treatment action campaign and the politics of HIV/AIDS*. Technical report, University of KwaZulu-Natal, Centre for Civil Society, Durban, South Africa.

Gauri, V. and Lieberman, E.S., 2006. Boundary institutions and HIV/AIDS policy in Brazil and South Africa. *Studies in Comparative International Development*, 41 (3), 47–73.

Girshick, R., 2004. Adopting institutional changes: HIV/AIDS and the changing institution of security. Paper prepared for the 44th Annual International Studies Association Convention, 25 February–1 March, Portland, Oregon.

Gómez, E.J., 2009. The politics of receptivity and resistance: how Brazil, India, China, and Russia strategically use the international health community in response to HIV/AIDS: a theory. *Global Health Governance*, III (1). Available from: http://blogs.shu.edu/ghg/files/2011/11/Gomez_The-Politics-of-Receptivity-and-Resistance_Fall-2009.pdf [accessed 15 April 2010].

Haven, B. and Patterson, A.S., 2007. The government-NGO disconnect: AIDS policy in Ghana. *In*: P.D. Siplon and P.G. Harris, eds. *The global politics of AIDS*. Boulder: Lynne Rienner, 65–86.

Heywood, M., 2009. South Africa's treatment action campaign: combining law and social mobilization to realize the right to health. *Journal of Human Rights Practice*, 1 (1), 14–36.

Iqbal, Z. and Zorn, C., 2010. Violent conflict and the spread of HIV/AIDS in Africa. *The Journal of Politics*, 72 (1), 149–162.

James, R. and Mullins, D., 2004. Supporting NGO partners affected by HIV/AIDS. *Development in Practice*, 14 (4), 574–585.

Jones, P., 2004. When 'development' devastates: donor discourses, access to HIV/AIDS treatment in Africa and rethinking the landscape of development. *Third World Quarterly*, 25 (2), 385–404.

Lieberman, E.S., 2009. *Boundaries of contagion: how ethnic politics have shaped government response to AIDS*. Princeton, NJ: Princeton University Press.

Mallouris, C., Caswell, G., and Bernard, E.J., 2010. How consultations by people living with HIV drive change and shape policies, programs and normative guidelines. *Global Health Governance*, IV (1).

May, C., 2007. Challenging global norms: the state, social costs, and legal action. *In*: R.L. Ostergard, ed. *HIV/AIDS and the threat to national and international security*, Global Issues Series. Houndmills: Palgrave Macmillan, 171–194.

McInnes, C., 2006. HIV/AIDS and security. *International Affairs*, 82 (2), 315–326.

de Mello e Souza, A., 2007. Defying globalization: effective self-reliance in Brazil. *In*: P.D. Siplon and P.G. Harris, eds. *The global politics of AIDS*. Boulder: Lynne Rienner, 37–63.

Ostergard, R.L., Jr., 2002. Politics in the hot zone: AIDS and national security in Africa. *Third World Quarterly*, 23 (2), 333–350.

Parkhurst, J.O. and Lush, L., 2004. The political environment of HIV: lessons from a comparison of Uganda and South Africa. *Social Science & Medicine*, 59 (9), 1913–1924.

Patel, P. and Tripodi, P., 2007. Linking HIV to peacekeepers. *In*: R.L. Ostergard, ed. *HIV/AIDS and the threat to national and international security*, Global Issues Series. Houndmills: Palgrave Macmillan, 107–124.

Patterson, A.S., 2006. *The politics of AIDS in africa*. Boulder: Lynne Rienner.

Paxton, N.A., 2010. *Learning to live?: examining differential international responses to HIV/AIDS*. Thesis (PhD). Harvard University, Cambridge, MA.

Peterson, S., 2002/2003. Epidemic disease and national security. *Security Studies*, 12 (2), 43–81.

Poku, N., 2002. Poverty, debt and Africa's HIV/AIDS crisis. *International Affairs*, 78 (3), 531–546.

Poku, N.K. and Sandkjaer, B., 2007. HIV/AIDS in the context of poverty: Africa's deadly predicament. *In*: R.L. Ostergard, ed. *HIV/AIDS and the threat to National and international security*, Global Issues Series. Houndmills: Palgrave Macmillan, 127–147.

Price-Smith, A.T., 2002. *The health of nations: infectious disease, environmental change, and their effects on national security and development.* Cambridge, MA: MIT Press.

Price-Smith, A.T., Tubin, M., and Ostergard, R.L., Jr. (2007). The decay of state capacity: HIV/AIDS and South Africa's national security. *In*: R.L. Ostergard, ed. *HIV/AIDS and the threat to national and international security*, Global Issues Series. Houndmills: Palgrave Macmillan, 241–260.

Putzel, J., 2004a. The global fight against AIDS: how adequate are the national commissions? *Journal of International Development*, 16 (8), 1129–1140.

Putzel, J., 2004b. The politics of action on AIDS: a case study of Uganda. *Public Administration and Development*, 24 (1), 19–30.

Putzel, J., 2006. A history of state action: the politics of AIDS in Uganda and Senegal. *In*: P. Denis and C. Becker, eds. *The HIV/AIDS epidemic in sub-Saharan Africa in a historical perspective.* Réseau sénégalais 'Droit, Éthique, Santé'. Available from: http://rds.refer.sn/sites/rds.refer.sn/IMG/pdf/16PUTZEL.pdf [accessed 15 April 2010].

Ramiah, I. and Reich, M.R., 2006. Building effective public–private partnerships: experiences and lessons from the African comprehensive HIV/AIDS partnerships (ACHAP). *Social Science & Medicine*, 63 (8), 397–408.

Robins, S., 2004. Long live Zackie, long live: AIDS activism, science and citizenship after apartheid. *Journal of Southern African Studies*, 30 (3), 651–672.

Roemer-Mahle, A., 2010. Business strategy and access to medicines in developing countries. *Global Health Governance*, IV (1). Available from: http://blogs.shu.edu/ghg/files/2011/11/Roemer-Mahler_Business-Strategy-and-Access-to-Medicines-in-Developing_Fall-2010.pdf [accessed 15 April 2010].

Rosen, S.P., 1987. Strategic implications of AIDS. *The National Interest*, 9, 64–73.

Schneider, H., 2002. On the fault-line: the politics of AIDS policy in contemporary South Africa. *African Studies*, 61 (1), 145–167.

Schneider, H. and Stein, J., 2001. Implementing AIDS policy in post-apartheid South Africa. *Social Science & Medicine*, 52 (5), 723–731.

Seckinelgin, H., 2008. *International politics of HIV/AIDS: global disease – local pain.* London: Routledge.

Sell, S.K., 2007. International institutions, intellectual property, and the HIV/AIDS pandemic. *In*: R.L. Ostergard, ed. *HIV/AIDS and the threat to national and international security*, Global Issues Series. Houndmills: Palgrave Macmillan, 148–170.

Shiffman, J., 2009. A social explanation for the rise and fall of global health issues. *Bulletin of the World Health Organization*, 87 (8), 608–613.

Siplon, P.D., 2005. AIDS and patriarchy: ideological obstacles to effective policy making. *In*: A.S. Patterson, ed. *The African state and the AIDS Crisis.* Aldershot: Ashgate, 17–36.

Smith, R.A. and Siplon, P.D., 2006. *Drugs into bodies: global AIDS treatment activism.* Westport, CT: Praeger.

Spiegel, P.B., 2004. HIV/AIDS among conflict-affected and displaced populations: dispelling myths and taking action. *Disasters*, 28 (3), 322–339.

Spiegel, P.B., *et al.*, 2007. Prevalence of HIV infection in conflict-affected and displaced people in seven sub-Saharan African countries: a systematic review. *Lancet*, 369 (9580), 2187–2195.

Strand, P., 2010. Making accountability work for the AIDS response. *Global Health Governance*, IV (1). Available from: http://blogs.shu.edu/ghg/files/2011/11/Strand_Making-Accountability-Work-for-the-AIDS-Response_Fall-2010.pdf [accessed 15 April 2010].

Stuckler, D., Basu, S., and McKee, M., 2010. Governance of mining, HIV and tuberculosis in Southern Africa. *Global Health Governance*, IV (1), 13.

Swidler, A., 2006. Syncretism and subversion in AIDS governance: how locals cope with global demands. *International Affairs*, 82 (2), 269–284.

Swidler, A. and Watkins, S.C., 2009. Teach a man to fish': the sustainability doctrine and its social consequences. *World Development*, 37 (7), 1182–1196.

Tantivess, S. and Walt, G., 2008. The role of state and non-state actors in the policy process: the contribution of policy networks to the scale-up of antiretroviral therapy in Thailand. *Health Policy and Planning*, 23 (5), 328–338.

de Waal, A., 2003. A disaster with no name: the HIV/AIDS pandemic and the limits of governance. *In*: G. Ellison, M. Parker and C. Campbell, eds. *Learning from HIV and AIDS.* Cambridge: Cambridge University Press, 238–267.

de Waal, A., 2010a. HIV/AIDS and the challenges of security and conflict. *The Lancet*, 375 (9708), 22–23.
de Waal, A., 2010b. Reframing governance, security and conflict in the light of HIV/AIDS: a synthesis of findings from the AIDS, security and conflict initiative. *Social Science & Medicine*, 70 (1), 114–120.
Weiss, M., 2006. Rejection as freedom? HIV/AIDS organizations and identity. *Perspectives on Politics*, 4 (4), 671–678.
White, J. and Morton, J., 2005. Mitigating impacts of HIV/AIDS on rural livelihoods: NGO experiences in sub-Saharan Africa. *Development in Practice*, 15 (2), 186–199.
Whiteside, A., 2002. Poverty and HIV/AIDS in Africa. *Third World Quarterly*, 23 (2), 313–332.
Whiteside, A., 2006. HIV/AIDS and development: failures of vision and imagination. *International Affairs*, 82 (2), 327–343.
Youde, J., 2005. The development of a counter-epistemic community: AIDS, South Africa, and international regimes. *International Relations*, 19 (4), 421–439.
Youde, J.R., 2007. *AIDS, South Africa, and the politics of knowledge*. Aldershot: Ashgate.

Descriptive representation and AIDS policy in South Africa

Evan S. Lieberman

The global AIDS pandemic raises key questions with respect to Pitkin's seminal concerns for the descriptive and substantive representation of diverse citizen interests. Specifically, are there 'group interests' for AIDS-related policies, and are they represented by political leaders? One might expect *all* politicians to prioritize a response to the global pandemic as a matter of public interest, especially in high prevalence countries. Alternatively, because recognizable sub-groups are affected differently, theories of representation imply that leader preferences should vary along these lines. The author explores the local political representation of AIDS-related interests within the context of the high prevalence, heterogeneous, and democratic society of South Africa. Through analysis of an original survey of the attitudes and preferences of local cancillors in Eastern Cape Province, he found that descriptive representation is associated with substantive representation: politicians express AIDS policy preferences in accordance with race- and gender-based interests, albeit in different ways.

Introduction

To date, most accounts of individual political leaders responding to the AIDS pandemic have tended toward one of two extremes: on the one hand, analysts working closely within AIDS policy circles have offered more voluntaristic accounts that emphasize the personal acumen or 'political will' of individual leaders.[1] For example, in a discussion of the early global governance response to HIV/AIDS, Merson (2006) explained, 'Despite its achievements, the Global Program on AIDS was unable to muster the necessary *political will* in donor and affected countries'; and Raviglione and Smith (2007), in the discussion of a tuberculosis (TB) control program, stated, 'These measures ultimately require political commitment and will, and in many countries, health is still not a top priority'. In a similar manner, when discussing the prospects for implementing highly active antiretroviral therapy in resource-poor settings, Farmer et al. (2001, p. 408) argued, 'These innovations require *political will* at high government levels'. Some analysts have tended to focus on the seemingly pathological former South African President Thabo Mbeki and his selected health ministers (Nattrass 2007) as examples of the autonomy of individual leaders.

On the other hand, political scientists and other social scientists studying the determinants of AIDS-related policies have tended toward the opposite end of the continuum, virtually dismissing the role of individual politicians and focusing instead on the structural and institutional pressures that shape policy-making. Such studies have argued that the content of policies can be predicted from a range of factors, such as level of economic development, HIV prevalence, levels of foreign funding, electoral cycles, patterns of ethnic relations, and other variables (e.g. Fourie 2006, Gauri and Lieberman 2006, Patterson 2006, Bor 2007, Strand 2007, Youde 2007, Lieberman 2009, Dionne 2011).

In this article, I explore a middle ground. I focus explicitly on the preferences of individual politicians, but I consider the factors that might help to explain why their views about AIDS policy vary even within the same institutional and structural contexts. Specifically, I consider their role as democratic *representatives*, which casts them in a quite different light from one in which they are described as isolated agents who may or may not possess 'political will'.

Particularly in diverse societies, Pitkin's (1967) notion of descriptive representation (p. 89) – the mirroring of the characteristics of the community within the representative body – is consequential because people tend to assume that those characteristics are good guides to the actions politicians will take in office. Importantly, however, she raises the question of whether in practice this leads to 'substantive' representation, or the actual representation of the diverse interests of the community. In numerous studies of the attitudes and behaviours of elected representatives in advanced industrialized countries, scholars have found evidence of substantive representation in legislative priorities according to individual characteristics such as race and gender. In a provocatively titled account of descriptive representation – 'Should blacks represent blacks and women represent women? A contingent "yes"' – Mansbridge (1999) argues that particularly for 'uncrystallized issues', the best representation may come from descriptive representatives.

To my knowledge no research has been conducted on the quality of representation for the problems of HIV, AIDS, or the closely associated TB epidemic.[2] These are leading causes of mortality and morbidity around the world, particularly in sub-Saharan Africa, and given the scope of the problems, they have not been considered along with more obviously distributive or targeted policy issues that are often the objects of analysis within studies of descriptive representation. Optimistically, one might like to think that major global public health issues would transcend 'group' interests. In other words, perhaps both citizens' and politicians' views about global public health and the health of their communities are shaped not by differences in terms of specific groups, but in terms of shared societal or even global concerns and priorities. If the latter were true, individual characteristics would not predict policy preferences. But in the complex reality of politics, citizens face many competing problems, and the threat of infectious disease clearly affects some groups of citizens more intensely than others. The question posed here is whether politicians themselves actually represent those views according to their own group characteristics, or if they simply reflect on the problems that face their constituencies, irrespective of group affiliations?

In this article, I focus explicitly on politicians. Specifically, I assess whether individual race and gender identities help to predict the infectious disease policy preferences of local politicians in the Eastern Cape Province of South Africa, potentially providing substantive representation of their own groups. As I discuss later, local cancillors provide an outstanding target for investigation, because they tend to live and work within close proximity to one another, facing the same local communities, and yet within diverse societies, they may be associated with different population sub-groups. Moreover, because local cancillors are called upon to be local problem solvers on a daily basis, their individual preferences and priorities are easily turned into action, in many ways unmediated by legislative or other institutions.

In the next section, I explain why citizens might have different intrinsic interests with respect to HIV and AIDS that vary along both race and gender lines, motivating an examination of whether such interests are differentially represented by local politicians. Subsequently, I describe the collection of data through an original survey of local cancillors, and present the main findings from various analyses of those data. I conclude by highlighting the theoretical and policy implications of this study. As a preview, I find that both race and gender *are* substantively represented by local cancillors, but in different ways, which ultimately cast a mixed light on the value of descriptive representation in this arena for the particular concerns of HIV, AIDS, and TB control.

Gender, race, and AIDS

Individual politicians, like individual citizens, can be described in terms of a virtually limitless number of personal characteristics, but as Pitkin (1967) notes, the notion of descriptive representation makes sense only in the context of politically relevant characteristics. In the context of AIDS in South Africa (the motivation for the choice of this location for study is discussed in the next section), the characteristics of both gender and race clearly merit investigation. Scholars studying descriptive representation in the USA and Europe have focused almost exclusively on these dimensions. And in South Africa, not only are these generally salient categories, but strong race- and gender-based political organizations have a longstanding history in the country: South Africa's history of institutionalized white supremacy is well known; moreover, women have routinely formed their own political organizations, such as the African National Congress (ANC) Women's league; and the Black Sash, a human rights organization founded by women to help other women and to protest the apartheid system of government.

Moreover, HIV prevalence varies substantially across gender and race lines within the country. The most authoritative survey of HIV prevalence finds that levels are much higher among women than men, particularly in the 25–29 age group, in which 32.7% of women were HIV-positive, as compared with male HIV prevalence of 15.7%. Nationwide, HIV prevalence for women was 13.6% and for men 7.9% (Shisana *et al.* 2009, p. 79). Starting in the early 1990s, scholars began writing about differential AIDS risk for women, and gender-targeted prevention strategies (e.g. de Bruyn 1992, Heise and Elias 1995) in developing countries, especially in Africa. In the specific case of South Africa, Albertyn (2003) argues that the AIDS epidemic has posed a distinctive threat to the prospects for gender equality. While there is no documented evidence of similar gender-based discrepancies in terms of TB prevalence, other factors, including the association of pregnancy with disease vulnerability (Bates *et al.* 2004, p. 268), contribute to the perception that TB also affects women disproportionately.

In other contexts, gender has been found to be an important predictor of politician preferences for particular public policies. For example, Poggione (2004) finds that female US state legislators are more liberal in their views on welfare policy; and in a study of village councils in West Bengal and Rajasthan states in India, Chattopadhyay and Duflo (2004) find that the gender composition of councils affected the types of public goods provided, specifically in line with gender-based preferences. In an analysis of the self-reported activities of 322 legislators in 12 American states, Thomas and Welch (1991) find that female state legislators were more attentive to women and family planning issues. And in a survey of Latin American legislators, Schwindt-Bayer (2006) finds substantial gender differences in attitudes toward women and children/family issues.

Drawing on these studies, it is reasonable to predict that in the case of HIV, AIDS, and perhaps to a lesser extent, TB, women might be more likely to perceive associated risks of and to express preferences for policies that target these diseases.

Similarly, race or ethnicity emerges in other contexts as an important determinant of policy preferences and priorities, and in racially divided societies (such as the USA), one would certainly be tempted to predict racially distinctive politician attitudes and behaviour. In a study of American legislators, Barrett (1995) finds distinctive race- and gender-based preferences for a range of policy issues. Particularly in the case of a stigmatized condition such as HIV, risk may be widely discussed in ethnic or racial terms (Cohen 1999, Lieberman 2009). In

South Africa, by 2008, 13.6% of Africans were HIV-positive, as compared with just 0.3% of whites and 1.7% of coloureds (Shisana *et al*. 2009, p. 79). Of course, in the South African context, the racial minorities (whites and coloureds) were previously advantaged politically, and still enjoy better socio-economic circumstances, so the normative implications of distributive and substantive representation are different than if those groups had been disadvantaged minorities. And yet, one of the cornerstone rationales for the value of descriptive representation is more diffuse legitimacy within the population, which itself is intrinsically valuable (Mansbridge 1999, p. 634).

Nonetheless, we should not always assume that gender or race will be robust predictors of policy preferences. As suggested, in the face of a substantial crisis, perhaps all leaders, irrespective of group characteristics, would perceive and prioritize objective dangers in the same way. Moreover, among women and among Africans, increasingly diverse socio-economic circumstances might dilute any sense of common interests: a wealthy, highly educated African male might have tastes more similar to that of a similarly wealthy and educated white woman than another African man who did not attend secondary school and lives in a shack. In short, one should not take for granted the primacy of any particular characteristic as a predictor of social salience (Connell 1987, Cornell and Hartman 1997), let alone policy preferences. Moreover, if one looks at the policy behaviour of three of South Africa's recent health ministers – Manto Tshabalala-Msimang (an African woman), Barbara Hogan (a white woman), and Aaron Motsoaledi (an African man) – experiences do not conform to theoretical expectations. Based on the discussion above, one should have expected the most aggressive response to AIDS from Tshabalala-Msimang, but without doubt, the opposite was true, as she helped lead a period of extreme AIDS denialism (Nattrass 2007). That said, it would be a mistake to generate inferences from just three politicians, who each emerged in very different political contexts and moments in history. A better approach is to engage in more systematic comparisons, to which I turn in the next section.

Research design

Do politicians with different group characteristics respond to similar circumstances in different ways? This is largely a descriptive question, and future research will need to more thoroughly examine causal pathways, as discussed in the conclusion. I seek to understand the extent of substantive representation for AIDS and TB by exploring the extent to which policy preferences and perceptions vary systematically in terms of group characteristics.

Along these lines, I chose to investigate *local* politicians for three key reasons. First, in recent years, local governments have been assigned increasing responsibility for service functions, including in the HIV sector, and yet to date, most research on the politics of policy-making has been at the national level. With just a few exceptions (e.g. Kelly and Van Donk 2009, Dionne 2010), local-level politicians have been under-studied in analyses of the response to HIV and this work helps to address that gap. Second, local politicians are useful to study for an analysis of policy preferences because within a relatively small area, a potentially large number of such politicians, at equal rank, and facing similar economic, political, and epidemiological conditions, can be studied systematically. This allows us to assess the effects of both constituency and individual characteristics. Third, local politicians tend to be easier to access than national politicians, who for various reasons tend to be less willing to complete the types of surveys routinely used to study policy preferences, such as the one used in this study.

I chose to study South Africa for several reasons, including the quite substantial prevalence of infectious diseases in that country, and increasing degree of policy decentralization – including in the area of HIV – which makes local cancillors an appropriate subject of investigation.

The country's history of heterodox AIDS policy responses in the wake of high HIV prevalence (Schneider 2002, Gauri and Lieberman 2006, Nattrass 2007) suggested that it might be a fruitful place to explore variation in policy preferences. The Eastern Cape was identified as a useful site for study as a diverse province – economically, racially, and in terms of local capacity. In terms of most human development indicators, it generally ranks in the middle of the nine South African Provinces. In 2008, HIV prevalence in the Eastern Cape was estimated at 9.0% for all persons, slightly lower than the national prevalence of 10.9% (Shisana et al. 2009, pp. xvi, 79).

The central source of data for the analyses presented below is an original survey of municipal local cancillors. While it is certainly true that much policy-making takes place in the offices of line ministries, such as departments of health, the motivation of the study was to better understand politicians who could plausibly address a very full range of problems. The initiative to focus on or prioritize a particular problem, such as AIDS or a related infectious disease, is truly meaningful only when a politician could plausibly address or choose to ignore that problem. That is, it would not be very interesting if the head of an AIDS commission said that AIDS was a priority. Along these lines, local cancillors are routinely called upon to help solve the myriad problems that citizens confront in their daily lives. Moreover, local cancillors are more than just legislators – they act as community leaders, assisting in the development of local programs and encouraging partnerships and constituent activities. Their own preferences are likely to mediate the implementation of government policies on the ground because they are likely to spend their time and political capital focused on priority issues, particularly as articulated by their political parties.

I employed a set of research assistants, including two American graduate students and three American undergraduates, along with two South African graduate students and one undergraduate. In total, three of the eight team members were male, and among the South Africans, two were black African, and native speakers of Xhosa, and the third was white and a native speaker of Afrikaans, but all three spoke fluent English. Because issues of race and language are politically sensitive in South Africa, our ability to form a team that contained a diverse membership provided good access to respondents.[3] We fielded a pen-and-paper survey of the attitudes and opinions of municipal cancillors that could be completed relatively quickly (in approximately 15 min). The survey questionnaire was developed in English, translated into the other local languages, Xhosa, and Afrikaans, back-translated into English, corrected and repeated until we were certain that the measurement instrument was consistent across languages.

The survey was fielded during the period June–August 2009. For each municipality, we began by contacting the speaker of the local council and requesting permission to distribute the survey to cancillors. We worked with the individual councils to identify the most effective strategy for distributing and retrieving the responses. Sometimes, cancillors filled out the survey prior to the start of a meeting, and at other times, they did this on their own time, within days of the survey being delivered to the council office. The cancillors returned the completed surveys to the secretary of the Speaker, who then forwarded the surveys to us. We provided a small, cash compensation to administrators in the speakers' offices for the extra work involved, and as an incentive for completing it, we told cancillors that all completed surveys would be entered in a lottery for a R1000 postal check cash prize, and this was paid to two cancillors at the conclusion of the survey.

We collected responses from 166 local cancillors across 11 municipalities in Cacadu and Amathole districts, and in the Nelson Mandela Metropolitan municipality. We achieved a response rate of 42.1% overall, and on average, 56.6% of cancillors in each municipality responded. Substantial political turmoil involving the recall of several top officials in Buffalo City Municipality during the summer of 2009 impeded the successful fielding of that survey. To a lesser extent, we also faced problems in Nelson Mandela – because we contacted the speaker of the council to obtain permission to field the survey, we learned that some cancillors feared the motivation of the survey was a test of 'political alliances'. Party in-fighting and protests shut down the municipal government in Sunday's River Valley which adversely affected the response rate. These issues notwithstanding, as discussed below, we attained a relatively representative sample relative in terms of the salient characteristics of the population.

The measurement and distribution of councillor policy preferences

Local councillor attitudes and policy preferences with respect to HIV, AIDS, and TB were measured along three dimensions: risk perception; policy prioritization; and support for specific policy proposals. When considering their responses, it is important to recall that councillors were not aware of our specific interest in HIV, AIDS, or infectious disease, and the survey asked questions about a wide range of topics that would be of concern to local governments. Councillors were told that the motivation for the study was an interest in the functioning of local democracy in South Africa, and the title on the survey form was, *Democracy in South Africa: Local Councillor Questionnaire*.

The distributions of responses are depicted in Figures 1–3. I measured risk perception by asking respondents to, 'Please rate the following risks in terms of how much they affect people…'. On a table that listed 16 different risks, they were asked to rate each one on a point scale as follows: 1, no risk; 2, minor risk; 3, moderate risk; 4, major risk; 5, extreme risk. Of all the risks considered, HIV was rated the most severe risk, with the mean response being 4.36 among councillors; theft and alcohol or drug abuse came second and third, with risk ratings of 4.13 and 4.08, followed by TB risk, which was rated 3.95. A full 88.9% of respondents rated the risk of HIV as being major or extreme, and 72.5% so rated the risk of TB. Thus,

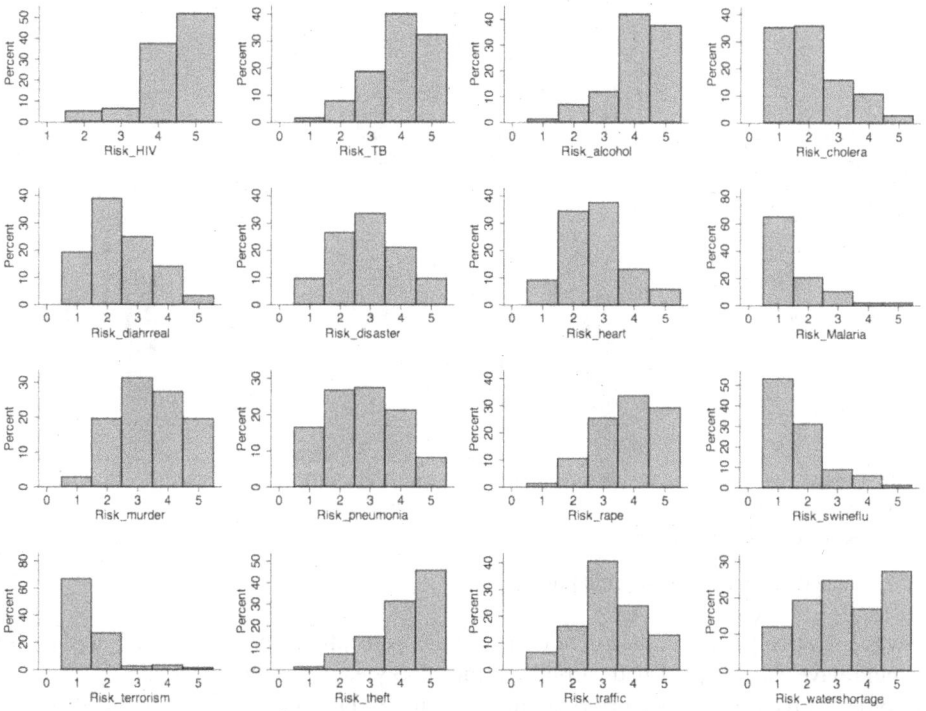

Figure 1. Distribution of councillor risk perceptions.

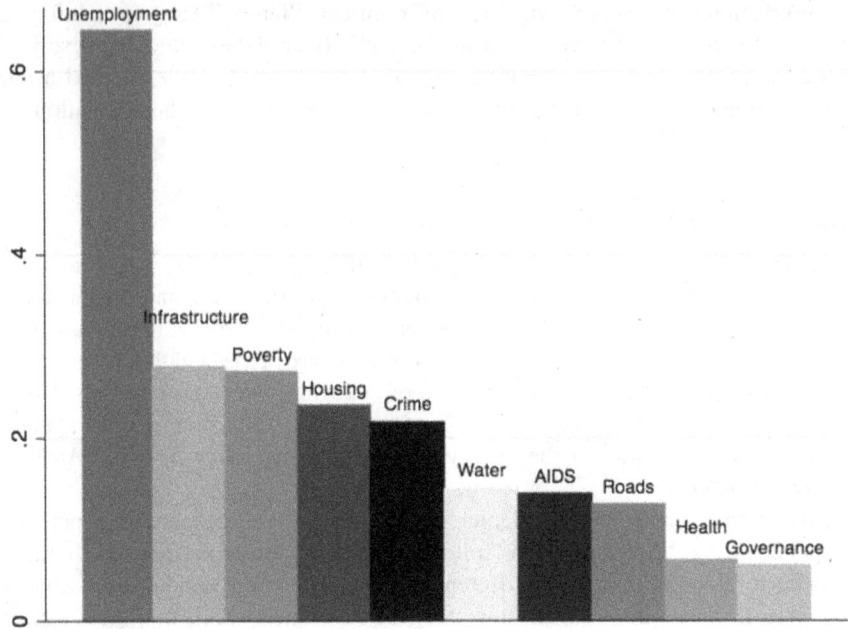

Figure 2. Councillor prioritization of AIDS as a leading problem.

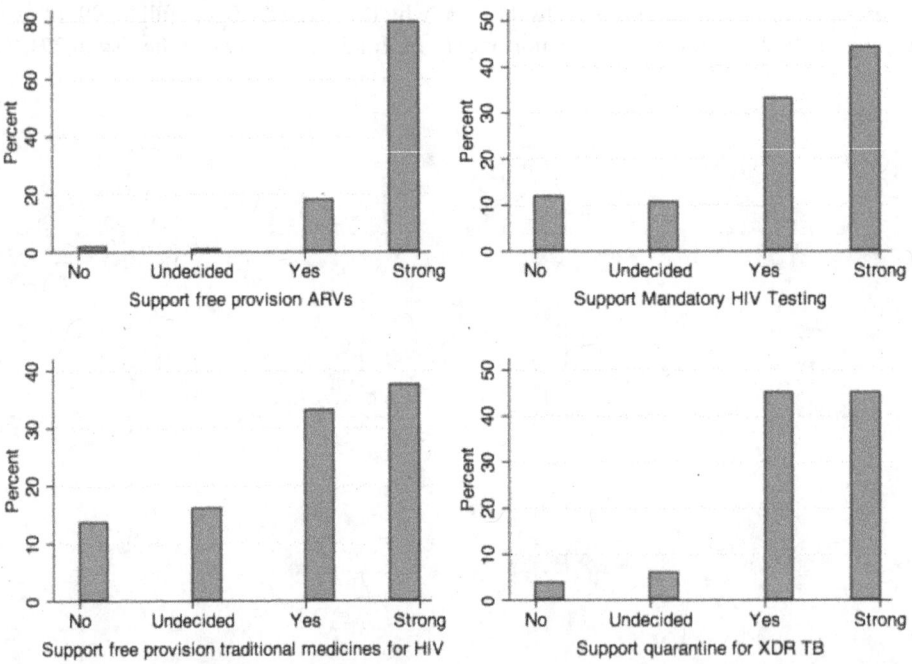

Figure 3. Councillor support for specific policies.

there was a relatively small degree of variation in risk perception, and certainly not to the degree one would have expected if I had carried out the survey earlier in the epidemic.

In order to measure policy prioritization, the survey began with an open-ended question, asking councillors, 'What are the three most important problems that you believe face people living in this municipality?' If they mentioned HIV or AIDS in any of their responses, I classified a dummy variable for AIDS prioritization as one; otherwise, it was coded zero. Only 13.9% mentioned HIV or AIDS as a priority, making it the seventh most mentioned priority among the councillors in our survey, following unemployment (64.5%), infrastructure (27.7%), poverty (27.1%), housing (23.5%), crime (21.7%), and water (14.5%). It is particularly interesting that although councillors, on average, rated the risk of HIV to be more severe than crime, the proportion of councillors identifying crime as a priority was more than 50% greater than the proportion that identified HIV or AIDS. The councillors surveyed generally represented poor municipalities and poor wards, and the issues surrounding poverty, security and basic services clearly took priority when compared with HIV and AIDS. And despite being a leading killer in a high prevalence area, TB was identified by just three councillors, making it one of the lowest expressed priorities. In light of the consensus around the high risk of being affected by HIV, AIDS, and TB, the relatively low prioritization as a policy issue is striking.

Along these lines, it is also important to highlight that councillors in our survey assigned a slightly lower priority to AIDS than citizens did more generally. On the 2008 round of the Afrobarometer survey, 21.1% of all respondents; and 16.7% of those from the Eastern Cape Province identified AIDS as one of the top three problems. However, it should be mentioned that the question wording was different – 'In your opinion, what are the most important problems facing this *country* that government should address?' Moreover, given that ours was not a representative sample of Eastern Cape councillors, and our respondents were from lower prevalence areas of the Eastern Cape, there is good reason to believe that overall, a similar share of local councillors identified AIDS as a priority that would have been found in an otherwise identical survey of citizens.

Finally, the survey asked questions about support for specific infectious disease-related public policies posed in terms of a list of other options. Specifically, the question asked, 'Which of the following policies and proposals do you support for *government action*? Please consider the likely costs and tradeoffs associated with any proposal. (Place an X in the column that best reflects your views.) The government should...' and for each policy proposal, the respondent was presented with a Likert scale, and could indicate one of four choices: No I do not support; I am undecided; Yes, I support; Yes, I strongly support.

The survey asked councillors to comment on four relevant policies: provide free antiretroviral (ARV) drugs to people who are HIV-positive; make HIV testing mandatory for everyone; provide free traditional remedies (like herbs or special foods) to people who are HIV-positive; and quarantine people with extremely multi-drug-resistant forms of TB (XDR TB). As shown in Figure 3, there was overwhelming support for the free provision of ARV's with 79.6% strongly supporting and another 17.9% supporting. While a large majority of respondents still supported the other three policies, there was less consensus around strong support, and the latter better indicates a willingness to take a leadership or aggressive role in promoting a particular policy. For mandatory testing, 44.4% strongly supported and 33.1% supported; for traditional medicines 37.4% strongly supported and 33.1% supported; and for XDR TB quarantines, 45.2% strongly supported and an additional 45.2% merely supported the proposal.

In the remainder of this article, I focus on exploring the determinants of variation in councillor attitudes and preferences, but it is worth reflecting on some of the key commonalities. To a large extent, the vast majority of local councillors *did* perceive a substantial risk from HIV, and agreed on several critical modalities for prevention and treatment. In a democratic context, one could imagine some conflicts over who benefits from public health spending, but when it comes to the free provision of ARV drugs, for example, this was not the case. Despite this, the vast majority of local councillors did not identify AIDS as one of their 'top priorities'. While

Dionne (2010) found similarly low levels of prioritization among village headmen in Malawi, in South Africa, infection levels are significantly higher, and general socio-economic conditions and infrastructure are better. Notwithstanding, local leaders, like citizens, placed many other basic needs higher on their lists of priorities. This is not necessarily a bad thing from the perspective of addressing the problems of infectious disease – for instance, better housing might reduce the transmission of TB; better job opportunities might reduce the extent of transactional sex that can lead to increased vulnerability to HIV transmission. But interested observers should be realistic about where AIDS stands in the hierarchy of quotidian concerns.

The characteristics of local councillors

In order to study the extent of substantive gender and race representation, I focus on the self-reported characteristics of the local councillors. Of particular interest, on both dimensions, I find an extremely high degree of descriptive representation, which is to say that the race and gender composition of the councillors in our sample comes quite close to mirroring the relative shares of groups within the population in those areas. (In Figure 4, I depict the relative distribution of the councillors in the survey sample in terms of race and gender.)

Although there are no specific enforcement mechanisms for the representation of women in the South African constitution, political parties have actively sought to attain gender parity, and have been increasingly successful in this regard since the 1994 elections (EISA 2009). In our sample, a full 53% of the respondents were female, which is exactly the share of female citizens counted in the 2001 census for the municipalities included in the study (author analysis of Census 2001 data).

In terms of race, South Africa has long used four racial categories, which persist to the present. According to the 2001 census, 71.5% of the residents in our study area were black African; 16.0% coloured; and 11.7% white, with a very small remainder (less than 1%) were Asian/Indian. While there are also no specific quotas for racial representation, the high degree of salience of race, in the context of a mixed electoral system at the local level that combines

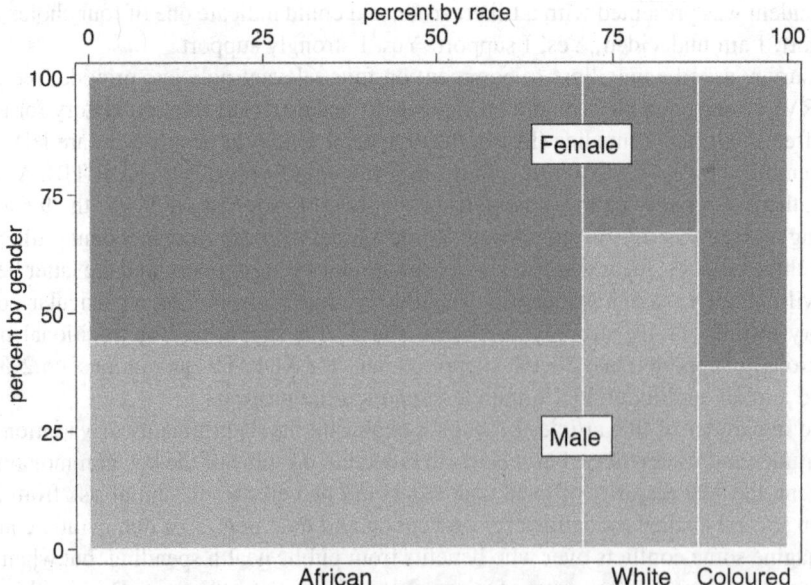

Figure 4. Race and gender composition of the local councillor survey.

proportional representation with single member wards (which themselves tend to be more racially homogeneous), has also led to strong descriptive representation. Within the sample, 69.9% of the councillors identified themselves as black African; 12.7% as coloured; and 16.3% as white.

Trying to understand the degree to which the race and gender of the councillors are actually associated with distinct policy preferences requires not only that I compare policy preferences across groups, but that I conduct 'fair' comparisons. For example, if the other characteristics of female councillors – for instance their age or level of education – are substantially different from those of their male counterparts, then gender group differences in policy preferences might reflect those other differences as much as they do the independent effect of gender. In some important ways, the South African case makes it quite difficult to establish such comparison, because the history of discrimination implies that the socio-economic circumstances of councillors varies substantially particularly by race group, and the internal composition of political parties are not reflective of the racial composition of the population more generally. A full 98% of the black African councillors were from the ANC party, while just 32% of the coloured and white councillors were from the ANC. Thus, it is extremely difficult to distinguish race from political party, which is a limitation of this study.

Other individual-level control variables, including level of education, age, extent of contact with external influences, personal experience with poverty, personal knowledge of someone who is HIV-positive, whether the councillor was elected to a ward (as compared with proportional representation) seat; and municipal-level characteristics, such as the racial fractionalization of the municipality and percent flush toilets are summarized in Table 1.

Analysis and discussion

I calculate the extent of substantively distinctive representation by race and gender by comparing average differences in responses along gender lines (reported in Table 2) and along race lines (reported in Table 3). For these analyses, I have re-scaled all of the outcome variables to a 0–1 range to facilitate meaningful comparisons.

In the first row of each of those tables, I simply report the differences in means between the test and control groups for each of the policy preference variables. These results do not account for heterogeneity of characteristics within groups. Again, for example in the case of race, this simple comparison of mean scores (evaluated for statistical significance with a *t*-test) does not control for the fact that on average, black councillors have less education than coloured and white councillors. On the other hand, such differences are still substantively meaningful in highlighting the reality of average group differences. In other words, if it is the case that race or gender are associated with other characteristics, this is likely recognized by voters, which in turn facilitates their ability to predict the likely preferences of that councillor even with little additional information.

In each of Tables 2 and 3, in rows 2–4, I present estimates of between-group differences using 'nearest-neighbour matching' (Abadie *et al.* 2004).[4] More generally, this technique is used to facilitate analysis of nonrandomized experiments as if the treatments had been randomly assigned. As compared with a simple comparison of means, this technique identifies one or more well-matched control cases for each treated case, and calculates differences on the outcome (here responses to survey questions) between the groups, adjusting for other differences that occur within the respective groups.

In these analyses, this technique allows me to generate descriptive inferences about how certain characteristics are associated with key policy preferences, independent of other individual traits. For example, by comparing the responses of female councillors with those of male

Table 1. Descriptive statistics.

Variable	Source/description	Obs.	Mean	Std. dev.	Min.	Max.
Female	DSLCS 2009 (0/1)	166	0.530	0.501	0	1
African	DSLCS 2009 (0/1)	166	0.699	0.460	0	1
Coloured	DSLCS 2009 (0/1)	166	0.127	0.333	0	1
White	DSLCS 2009 (0/1)	166	0.163	0.370	0	1
Risk HIV	DSLCS 2009 (five-point scale)	162	0.840	0.202	0.25	1
Risk TB	DSLCS 2009 (five-point scale)	157	0.737	0.242	0	1
AIDS priority	DSLCS 2009 (0/1 – if mentioned as one top 3 'most important problems that you believe face people living in this municipality')	166	0.139	0.347	0	1
Support free ARVs	DSLCS 2009 (four-point scale)	162	0.918	0.186	0	1
Support mandatory HIV testing	DSLCS 2009 (four-point scale)	160	0.700	0.337	0	1
Support traditional medicine for AIDS	DSLCS 2009 (four-point scale)	163	0.648	0.346	0	1
Support quarantine for people with XDR TB	DSLCS 2009 (four-point scale)	155	0.772	0.251	0	1
Age	DSLCS 2009 (1, 20–39; 2, 40–59; 3, 60+)	162	2.068	0.641	1	3
Education	DSLCS 2009 (2, not completed high school; 3, completed high school; 4, some university/college; 5, completed university/college)	163	3.479	1.119	2	5
Personal knowledge of people who have died of AIDS last year	DSLCS 2009 (0/1)	165	0.891	0.313	0	1
Poverty index	DSLCS 2009: three-point scale based on questions about personal experiences with hunger, informal housing, and lack of flush toilet	165	1.782	1.143	0	3
External influence	DSLCS 2009: average level of influence of donors, experts, and civil society organizations, based on self-reported consultations	161	1.665	0.680	1	3
Ward councillor	DSLCS 2009 (0/1)	165	0.570	0.497	0	1
Percent households with flush toilets in councillor constituency	Statistics South Africa 2009. For ward councillors, used wards; for PR councillors, used municipality	164	0.491	0.322	0.001	0.995
Race fractionalization 2001	Statistics South Africa 2009 (author calculated Herfindahl index)	166	0.393	0.213	0.006	0.626

Note: DSLCS 2009: democracy in South Africa Local Councillor Study (author).

councillors who are otherwise extremely similar in many important respects, I am able to isolate the how gender is associated with councillor attitudes – which is the key concern for measuring the extent of substantive representation. To be clear, this is a descriptive analysis, and I am not attempting to make *causal* inferences about the effects of race or gender. In the second row of each table, I match on only a single trait – race in the case of the gender comparison and gender in the case of the race comparison. In the third row, I add a set of individual-level controls,

Table 2. Gender differences in AIDS policy preferences.

Comparison: female vs. male	HIV risk	TB risk	AIDS priority	Support free ARVs	Support mandatory HIV testing	Support traditional medicine for AIDS	Support XDR TB quarantine
No controls (t-test)	0.073** (0.031)	0.065* (0.038)	0.068 (0.054)	0.031 (0.029)	0.115* (0.053)	0.080# (0.054)	0.035 (0.040)
NN matching on race	0.070* (0.031)	0.070# (0.039)	0.066 (0.053)	0.025 (0.029)	0.091# (0.052)	0.047 (0.052)	0.040 (0.040)
NN matching on race, minimal controls	0.062# (0.032)	0.069# (0.040)	0.087 (0.056)	0.028 (0.027)	0.075 (0.057)	0.031 (0.054)	0.069# (0.042)
NN matching on race, many controls	0.071* (0.034)	0.084* (0.042)	0.067 (0.058)	0.028 (0.029)	0.080 (0.058)	0.053 (0.053)	0.059 (0.042)

Notes: NN, using 'nearest-neighbour' matching with inverse variance bias correction in rows 2–4. Size of standard errors is in parentheses. Minimal controls: age, poverty history, and ward councillor; many controls also include education, personal HIV, flush toilet share, and race fractionalization.
*$p < 0.05$.
**$p < 0.01$.
#$p < 0.10$.

Table 3. Race differences in AIDS policy preferences.

Comparison: black Africans vs. whites and coloureds	HIV risk	TB risk	AIDS priority	Support free ARVs	Support mandatory HIV testing	Support traditional medicine for AIDS	Support XDR TB quarantine
No controls (t-test)	0.041 (0.035)	−0.041 (0.042)	0.084# (0.057)	0.029 (0.031)	0.126* (0.056)	0.246** (0.000)	−0.105** (0.043)
NN matching on gender	0.030 (0.034)	−0.057 (0.041)	0.080 (0.055)	0.024 (0.031)	0.116* (0.057)	0.228** (0.060)	−0.109** (0.040)
NN matching on gender, minimal controls	0.046 (0.041)	−0.094* (0.047)	0.047 (0.066)	0.056 (0.035)	0.100 (0.069)	0.128* (0.062)	−0.123** (0.043)
NN matching on gender, many controls	−0.006 (0.039)	−0.070 (0.049)	0.075 (0.069)	0.021 (0.036)	0.092 (0.074)	0.174** (0.065)	−0.101* (0.049)

Notes: NN, using 'nearest-neighbour' matching with inverse variance bias correction in rows 2–4. Size of standard errors is in parentheses. Minimal controls: age, poverty history, and ward councillor; many controls also include education, personal HIV, flush toilet share, and race fractionalization.
*$p < 0.05$.
**$p < 0.01$.
#$p < 0.10$.

including age, a measure of the councillor's personal experiences with poverty, and a dummy variable for whether the councillor is a ward councillor. Finally, in the fourth row, I also add controls for level of education, personal knowledge of someone who died of AIDS last year, the percentage of households in that councillor's constituency that have flush toilets, and the degree of racial heterogeneity or fractionalization of the municipality. In these analyses, analytic control is achieved through identification of control cases that are closest to the treatment case in terms of values on these other variables, and by weighting the results according to the quality of the matches.

The results demonstrate quite clearly a few gender- and race-based differences in councillor responses to the survey. However, the patterns are themselves quite distinctive across cleavages. Women clearly perceive the risks of HIV and TB as being more severe relative to their male counterparts; and despite the fact that inter-racial differences in HIV prevalence were orders of magnitude higher than with respect to gender, there were no statistically significant differences across race lines. And in the case of perceived TB risk, black African councillors actually reported lower levels of perceived risk than white and coloured councillors.

In terms of responses to the open-ended question about municipal priorities, both female and African councillors were more likely than men and whites/coloureds respectively to identify AIDS, but in neither case was this finding consistently robust at conventional levels of statistical significance.[5] There was also no substantial difference between groups in terms of support for the free provision of ARV drugs to people who are HIV-positive. In this case, there was so much consensus that this was a good policy idea among the entire sample of respondents that it was frankly implausible that I would find substantial differences in terms of race and/or gender. Nonetheless, it is worth reflecting that white and coloured councillors in this area could plausibly have opposed free provision, given that white and coloured constituents would be extremely unlikely to directly benefit, and yet, they supported this as a general policy.

In terms of other disease-related policy preferences, a few key findings stand out: first, preferences vary more widely along race lines than along gender lines. Quite clearly, black Africans are substantially *more* supportive of the proposal to provide free traditional remedies to people who are HIV-positive. In general, Africans disproportionately utilize traditional doctors and remedies, and this finding reflects this general tendency. Alternatively, Africans are much *less* supportive of quarantining individuals with multi-drug-resistant TB, which likely reflects both a concern that such a policy would more likely restrict the personal liberties of members of their group, and a general resistance to any form of incarceration, given the bitter history of detentions for black Africans in the country. That said, black Africans favour mandatory testing to a greater extent than councillors from other race groups, but with greater analytic control – matching on a larger number of covariates – the magnitude of differences shrinks, while the size of the standard error increases. Women are more supportive than are men of all of the policy proposals, but only in the case of support for mandatory HIV testing are the results sufficiently robust across (three of four) model estimates. This finding further highlights female councillors' distinctive concern for HIV status.

Are these patterns unique to HIV and AIDS? Or do they simply reflect more general differences in risk perceptions and policy preferences or even different styles of answering questions along gender and race lines? In Table 4, I report nearest-neighbour matching estimates of gender and race group comparisons for a wider range of questions about risk perception (murder, diarrheal disease, traffic accidents) and support for various policies (harsher prison terms, extending opportunities to people from historically disadvantaged groups, and allocating more resources to water delivery/quality). The findings of this analysis suggest that leader responses were specific to the particular issues and questions addressed on the survey. While it is true that female councillors generally reported higher perception of risks, this was not the case for traffic accidents,

Table 4. Gender and race effects on risk perception and policy preferences, not AIDS-related.

Comparisons	Risk murder	Risk diarrheal disease	Risk traffic accidents	Risk water shortage	Support harsher prison term	Support opportunity to historically disadvantaged	Support allocating more resources to water delivery
Gender (NN matching on race, many controls)	0.382* (0.182)	0.331# (0.176)	0.020 (0.181)	0.345 (0.229)	0.037 (0.051)	0.186 (0.139)	−0.005 (0.079)
Race (NN matching on gender, many controls)	−0.170 (0.202)	−0.357 (0.223)	−0.573** (0.214)	−0.245 (0.268)	0.017 (0.064)	0.348* (0.172)	0.025 (0.101)

Note: NN, using 'nearest-neighbour' matching with inverse variance bias correction. Size of standard errors is in parentheses. Matching on: age, education, poverty history, ward councillor, flush toilet share, and race fractionalization.
*$p < 0.05$.
**$p < 0.01$.
#$p < 0.10$.

and the differences were not statistically significant in the case of water shortages. Race proved to be a statistically significant predictor of perceived risk of traffic accidents (many fewer Africans drive relative to the size of their group as compared with whites), and perhaps not surprisingly, African councillors were more supportive of redistributive policies to historically disadvantaged groups – a phrase that generally connotes black African-oriented redistribution, but is sometimes used for gender- and class-based redistribution in the South African context. Despite wide variation in responses to the policy proposals in the sample, there was no systematic difference in support for the other policy proposals along race lines.

These findings suggest that there are indeed substantive implications for descriptive representation with respect to HIV and AIDS, at least from an attitudinal standpoint. I cannot, from this analysis alone, draw any conclusions about what councillors actually do within their constituencies, or whether the policies and practices of their respective councils would be different if they had been racially homogeneous or less gender-balanced in composition. But if we proceed with the assumption that at least to an extent, actions follow perceptions and preferences, there is good reason to believe that the high levels of descriptive representation in local government leads to the substantive representation of the diversity of views on infectious disease control, and may explain why some politicians appear to have more 'political will' on the issue than others.

Conclusions and future research

This study sheds some important light on the nature of descriptive representation in the high HIV prevalence, heterogeneous democracy of South Africa. In line with knowledge that women tend to face greater personal danger from the epidemic, and shoulder the lion's share of care giving for sick members of households and communities, I found that female councillors reported higher levels of perceived HIV and TB risk. But those differences did not translate into gender-specific preferences for action. Meanwhile, substantial differences across race lines in terms of what councillors believe ought to be *done* was not associated with differential risk perceptions across race groups, despite exponential differences in group HIV prevalence. To an extent, the null finding in terms of differences in risk perception across race groups is due to the fact that the vast majority of councillors perceive HIV to be a relatively high-risk problem in the areas they work. But the finding is also consistent with the proposition put forth in Lieberman (2009) that in the context of a stigmatized condition, there may be greater risk denial on the part of high prevalence race or ethnic groups, owing to perceived shame of association.

What are the substantive implications of such patterns of representation? This study suggests that at the very least, along the cleavages of race and gender, citizens' diverse interests with respect to infectious disease are being expressed within local legislatures. And to the extent that good democratic governance requires full consideration of the needs and preferences of citizens, descriptive representation facilitates such outcomes. Citizens can find representation of at least some of their interests merely by electing leaders who, to an extent, look like themselves – whether they do this through direct elections, or through institutions such as those in South Africa, which have provided a high degree of descriptive representation. Through processes of deliberation, better policies may be enacted and implemented because democratic representatives have the opportunities to discuss and to engage a range of views.

On the other hand, the flip side of the representation of diverse interests is the heightened potential for conflict. A long line of scholarship has highlighted the pathologies associated with, for example, ethnic diversity when it comes to policy-making. Moreover, as Diamond (1990) has argued, one of the paradoxes of democracy is that the reconciliation of conflicting interests can make governance difficult. Macro-level studies of AIDS policy-making have not found a strong association between level of democracy and quality of response, and it remains to be explored whether regimes characterized by a high degree of descriptive representation do better than those that lack such qualities.

To be certain, the empirical project presented here is a modest one, exploring the expressed preferences of just 166 local councillors in a single South African province. But it is the first systematic attempt to understand why elected local politicians might have different preferences concerning a leading source of mortality and morbidity. In so doing it provides additional evidence concerning the link between descriptive and substantive representation as well as useful insights about the attitudes of political leaders, which in other contexts have been treated rather ambiguously as instances of 'political will'. The findings remind us that politicians do not simply act as free agents. In a democratic context, they also serve as representatives of various subgroups within society. Future research will be needed to examine why some characteristics and not others serve as useful heuristics for representing citizen interests, and what exactly leads politicians to hold particular views. (For example, is it their shared experiences as members of a 'group'? Calculations about what their group needs? Or perceptions of what their group wants?)

Given that South Africa remains the epicentre of the global AIDS pandemic and that local governments are increasingly being asked to do more suggests that the subject of analysis is substantively important. Moreover, given the extremely paltry base of knowledge, this work is necessary to establish a preliminary understanding of problem perception, prioritization, and attitudes toward related policies. To build on this, much larger samples of leaders from different places and with different responsibilities ought to be studied; other measures of policy preferences and behaviour need to be developed; and other research designs, including survey and field experiments, or even repeated surveys, are needed to better identify the determinants of what politicians think and what they do.

Acknowledgements

I gratefully acknowledge financial support from Princeton's Grand Challenges fund and the Decker Fund, and excellent research assistance from Irfan Kherani, Erin Lin, Qiong Qiu, and Shivani Sud, Gcobani Qambela, Estelle Prinsloo, and Siyabonga-ka-Phindile Yonzi. Gwyneth McClendon managed the survey of municipal councillors described herein. Thanks to Lin, McClendon, John Gerring, Jessica Grody, Kent Buse, Dennis Altman, and two anonymous reviewers for comments.

Notes

1. In general, the term 'political will' has not been well conceptualized or defined, but I assume that the term is used to connote an interest in how aggressively individual politicians respond to the policy issue of interest (infectious disease control). More recently, Post *et al.* (2010) and Fox *et al.* (2011) have offered useful discussions about how to define and analyse 'political will'.
2. Discussed here as part of the AIDS epidemic because in sub-Saharan Africa, more than 70% of HIV-positive individuals are co-infected with TB and co-infection can accelerate disease progression and make treatment less effective (Bates *et al.* 2004, p. 271).
3. *Protection of human subjects*: because all respondents were publicly elected officials, who routinely speak about these questions in their work and for public audiences, Princeton University granted this project an exemption from full IRB review.
4. I obtain largely similar results using ordinary least squares, logit, and ordered logit estimation using the minimal controls specifications. However, given the relatively small sample size, the statistical significance of the estimates is more sensitive to alternate model specifications. Estimates of the effects of

gender are robust to inclusion of a dummy variable for ANC party membership. In the nearest neighbour matching estimates, no more than 25 observations were excluded owing to the absence of suitable matches.
5. Because this was a dichotomous outcome, in which a relatively small share of all respondents answered affirmatively, it stands to reason that these findings might have been statistically significant in a larger sample.

References

Abadie, A., *et al.*, 2004. Implementing matching estimators for average treatment effects in Stata. *Stata Journal*, 4 (3), 290–311.

Albertyn, C., 2003. Contesting democracy: HIV/AIDS and the achievement of gender equality in South Africa. *Feminist Studies*, 29 (3), 595–615.

Barrett, E.J., 1995. The policy priorities of African American women in state legislatures. *Legislative Studies Quarterly*, 20 (2), 223–247.

Bates, I., *et al.*, 2004. Vulnerability to malaria, tuberculosis, and HIV/AIDS infection and disease. Part 1: determinants operating at individual and household level. *The Lancet Infectious Diseases*, 4 (5), 267–277.

Bor, J., 2007. The political economy of AIDS leadership in developing countries: an exploratory analysis. *Social Science & Medicine*, 64 (8), 1585–1599.

de Bruyn, M., 1992. Women and aids in developing countries: the XIIth international conference on the social sciences and medicine. *Social Science & Medicine*, 34 (3), 249–262.

Chattopadhyay, R. and Duflo, E., 2004. Impact of reservation in Panchayati Raj: evidence from a nationwide randomised experiment. *Economic and Political Weekly*, 39 (9), 979–986.

Cohen, C.J., 1999. *The boundaries of blackness: AIDS and the breakdown of black politics*. Chicago: University of Chicago Press.

Connell, R., 1987. *Gender and power: society, the person, and sexual politics*. Cambridge: Polity Press in association with B. Blackwell.

Cornell, S.E. and Hartmann, D., 1997. *Ethnicity and race: making identities in a changing world*. Thousand Oaks, CA: Pine Forge Press.

Diamond, L., 1990. Three paradoxes of democracy. *Journal of Democracy*, 1 (3), 48–60.

Dionne, K.Y., 2010. *Study of AIDS and governance in Malawi*. Doctoral dissertation (PhD). UCLA.

Dionne, K.Y., 2011. The role of executive time horizons in state response to AIDS in Africa. *Comparative Political Studies*, 44 (1), 55–77.

Electoral Institute for the Sustainability of Democracy in South Africa (EISA), 2009. *Women's representation quotas*. Johannesburg. Available from: http://www.eisa.org.za/WEP/souquotas.htm [accessed 12 December 2011].

Farmer, P., *et al.*, 2001. Community-based approaches to HIV treatment in resource-poor settings. *Lancet*, 358 (9279), 404–409.

Fourie, P., 2006. *The political management of HIV and AIDS in South Africa: one burden too many?* Houndmills: Palgrave Macmillan.

Fox, A., *et al.*, 2011. Conceptual and methodological challenges to measuring political commitment to respond to HIV. *Journal of the International AIDS Society*, 14 (Suppl. 2), 1–13.

Gauri, V. and Lieberman, E., 2006. Boundary politics and government responses to HIV/AIDS in Brazil and South Africa. *Studies in Comparative International Development*, 41 (3), 47–73.

Heise, L.L. and Elias, C., 1995. Transforming AIDS prevention to meet women's needs: a focus on developing countries. *Social Science & Medicine*, 40 (7), 931–943.

Kelly, K. and Van Donk, M., 2009. Local-level responses to HIV/AIDS in South Africa. *In*: P. Rohleder, ed. *HIV/AIDS in South Africa 25 years on: psychosocial perspectives*. New York: Springer, 135–154.

Lieberman, E.S., 2009. *Boundaries of contagion: how ethnic politics have shaped government responses to AIDS*. Princeton: Princeton University Press.

Mansbridge, J., 1999. Should blacks represent blacks and women represent women? A contingent 'yes'. *The Journal of Politics*, 61 (3), 628–657.

Merson, M.H., 2006. The HIV/AIDS pandemic at 25: the global response. *New England Journal of Medicine*, 354 (23), 2414–2417.

Nattrass, N., 2007. *Mortal combat: AIDS denialism and the struggle for antiretrovirals in South Africa*. Scottsville: University of KwaZulu-Natal Press.

Patterson, A.S., 2006. *The politics of AIDS in Africa*. Boulder, CO: Lynne Rienner.

Pitkin, H., 1967. *The concept of political representation*. Berkeley: University of California Press.

Poggione, S., 2004. Exploring gender differences in state legislators' policy preferences. *Political Research Quarterly*, 57 (2), 305–314.

Post, L.A., Raile, A.N.W., and Raile, E.D., 2010. Defining political will. *Politics and Policy*, 38 (4), 653–676.

Raviglione, M.C. and Smith, I.M., 2007. XDR tuberculosis – implications for global public health. *New England Journal of Medicine*, 356 (7), 656–659.

Schneider, H., 2002. On the fault-line: the politics of AIDS policy in contemporary South Africa. *African Studies*, 61 (1), 145–167.

Schwindt-Bayer, L.A., 2006. Still supermadres? Gender and the policy priorities of Latin American legislators. *American Journal of Political Science*, 50 (3), 570–585.

Shisana, O., et al., 2009. *South African national HIV prevalence, incidence, behaviour and communication survey, 2008: a turning tide among teenagers?* Cape Town, South Africa: HSRC Press.

Statistics South Africa, 2009. *Population census 2001*. Available from: http://www.statssa.gov.za/ [accessed 1 April 2009].

Strand, P., 2007. Comparing AIDS governance: a research agenda on responses to the AIDS epidemic. *In*: N. Poku, A. Whiteside, and B. Sandkjaer, eds. *AIDS and governance*. Aldershot, UK; Burlington, VT: Ashgate, 217–236.

Thomas, S. and Welch, S., 1991. The impact of gender on activities and priorities of state legislators. *The Western Political Quarterly*, 44 (2), 445–456.

Youde, J.R., 2007. *AIDS, South Africa, and the politics of knowledge*. Burlington, VT: Ashgate.

Public opinion as leadership disincentive: exploring a governance dilemma in the AIDS response in Africa

Per Strand

There is increasing emphasis in global declaration on the need to get politics right in the response to AIDS, particularly in terms of strengthening accountable leadership. However, in the worst affected countries in sub-Saharan Africa, such governance prescriptions introduce political concerns that are not well understood. In a context of the neo-patrimonial governance that characterises African democracies, the paper analyses data from the Afrobarometer on public opinions on AIDS in 20 countries to identify and explore the governance dilemma that leaders face when they are expected to show strong leadership on an issue that is low on the public political agenda. By identifying country-level correlates and individual-level determinants of the strong opinion on AIDS that is held by a minority, the paper suggests how public opinion for an effective response can be mobilised in ways that are politically sustainable.

Introduction

The countries in sub-Saharan Africa are by far the worst affected by the global AIDS epidemic. By the latest count, the region holds two-thirds of the world's HIV-positive people and some of the countries have 'hyperendemic HIV' with over 15% of the adult population infected (UNAIDS 2010). At such an alarming scale, AIDS leads to aggregate effects such as reduced life expectancy and increased poverty (Poku 2005). Advances in development, human rights and gender equality that took decades to accomplish have been lost (Whiteside 2007). In order to reverse the epidemic and regain lost ground in terms of development the response to HIV and AIDS has to be comprehensive and long-term, with human rights-based strategies and developmental goals that go far beyond the parameters of a strict public health-oriented approach (Irurzun-Lopez and Poku 2005). The success of such a broad and multi-dimensional approach will to no small degree depend on the quality of political governance in the State.

Policy-makers at the highest levels are increasingly recognising that political factors are central to an effective response. The most recent United Nations Declaration on the global effort against HIV and AIDS acknowledges that 'poorly coordinated and transaction-heavy responses and lack of proper governance and financial accountability impede progress' (United Nations 2011, paragraph 45). An intensified response should therefore be defined by 'decisive, inclusive and accountable leadership' by governments in order to reach the agreed upon targets for HIV prevention, AIDS treatment and care and support services (United Nations 2011, paragraph 50). The normative political instruments for the global AIDS response are correct in emphasising the need for accountability. However, there are complexities linked to such a governance prescription that are not yet well understood, complexitites that may in fact provide disincentives for strong political leadership of the response to AIDS.

The nature of public opinion on HIV and AIDS in sub-Saharan Africa makes this point very clearly. In a democratic political system, public opinion would leverage electoral pressure on politicians to ensure an effective response under three conditions. Firstly, the response to AIDS must be a political priority for voters. People's general concerns with AIDS will have little political effect if they do not think that AIDS is one of the most important current political issues that government should address. Secondly, public opinion must mainly be critical of government's past performance in the response; it would present no incentive for stronger action if governments are only applauded for their efforts. The third condition is that general elections are used as a mechanism to sanction under-performing governments. Even critical popular opinion will have little political impact if people's electoral preferences are not based on their scrutiny of government performance. Neither of these three conditions can be assumed for the region as a whole, or even in the countries that are worst affected with hyperendemic HIV. Previous research on public opinion on AIDS in Africa has shown that the first condition does not hold: only a minority of voters in the region think that HIV and AIDS should be a top priority for their respective governments (Mattes 2004, Whiteside et al. 2004). On the basis of that research, Alex De Waal argues that the ballot box will not be an effective accountability mechanism to leverage stronger political leadership on AIDS. Instead, he continues, under-performance on HIV prevention will persist 'because [governments] haven't been required to succeed. When African and international electorates punish their leaders for this failure, we can expect progress' (2006, p. 123).

The purpose of this paper is to identify the governance dilemma that arises when an effective response to HIV and AIDS demands that government prioritises resources and provide leadership in ways that have little support in public opinion. The paper will provide an updated and comprehensive set of public opinion data on AIDS from 20 countries in sub-Saharan Africa, as collected by the Afrobarometer.[1] On the basis of this data, the paper will introduce the notion of an 'AIDS constituency' as the group of prospective voters that is most likely to allow their opinions on AIDS to influence their electoral choice. In an effort to identify patterns in the data, the paper will explore country-level correlates with public opinion and then seek to identify individual-level characteristics that make individuals more likely to be part of the AIDS constituency. On the basis of these analyses the paper will discuss what strategies and interventions may be more successful in trying to mobilise public opinion on AIDS to a point that electoral politics become an effective incentive for stronger government leadership in the AIDS response.

Public opinion and accountability in African politics

The level of correspondence between government policy and public opinion relates to three principles that, while they are insufficient as a definition of democracy, are central to democratic governance: representation, responsiveness and vertical accountability, i.e. the power of voters to punish under-performing governments in elections (Schmitter 2005). The normative weight of these principles vary somewhat between alternative conceptions of democracy and good governance, but most would agree that a democracy is of a higher quality if it is representative of the public's values and policy priorities, if it is responsive to strong and sustained shifts in public opinion and if politicians and parties can be held accountable for poor performance through the electoral process (Diamond and Morlino 2005). While such general normative sentiments seem uncontroversial, an effective response to AIDS in sub-Saharan Africa may be in conflict with all three of these principles. Whether or not this is the case depends on the nature of public opinion on HIV and AIDS.

Firstly, the principle of representation would support an effective response only if the majority of people, or at least a considerable minority, agreed with the scale of the government's effort and the nature of the interventions. Lacking such support, one would hope that the government nevertheless would be able to sustain the response. Secondly, a government that has adopted a national policy based on the global guidelines of a human rights-based approach should not be responsive to public sentiments that discriminate against people who are HIV positive or due to their sexual orientation. Finally, the prospects of a misinformed and prejudiced voting public punishing a government that is making good progress in the response is a disincentive for any government to act decisively in opposition to adverse public opinion. These political dynamics would help explain why previous research has been unable to establish a link between effective responses and democratic characteristics of political governance in African countries (Bor 2007, Strand et al. 2008).

As a way of contextualising the public opinion data that will be presented and analysed further below, the next two sections will introduce two discourses on political governance in Africa that discuss the rationale for electoral choice and the likelihood of vertical accountability.

What determines electoral choice in Africa?

Michael Bratton and his colleagues identify five theories that claim to answer that question: *social structure* in terms of demographic factors, *cultural values* that define political loyalties, *institutional influences* such as membership or loyalty to a political party, *cognitive awareness* in terms of formal education and interest in politics and *performance evaluations* of past government performance (Bratton et al. 2005, pp. 34–43). The discourse has debated whether it is culture or evaluation that ultimately decide electoral choice. A nuanced perspective that avoids a simplistic choice between the two theories has been suggested by Dan Posner. In his seminal study of ethnic politics in Zambia, Posner argues that to the extent individual voters support ethnic parties they do so mainly for rational and not emotional reasons: 'it is the information ethnicity is assumed to convey about likely patterns of patronage distribution – not atavism or tradition – that explains why it plays such an important role in Zambian political life' (2006, p. 91, see also Bratton et al. 2011). The rationale for such behaviour lies in the neo-patrimonial features of the African democracies (Hyden 2006). Neo-patrimonialism is a system of informal governance that merges 'traditional' and ethnically defined hierarchies of power and systems of patronage with formal 'modern' processes and institutions in the democratic state. Once they have gained access, political elites and governing parties use public resources as means to reinforce ethnic boundaries, thus making the 'ethnic vote' a 'rational' option for voters to secure resources for themselves. This form of governance is by no means unique to Africa but its influence is relatively strong due to the weakness of governance norms and processes that are rule-bound and universal in character. While the detrimental effects of this form of governance for development is well established, Evan Lieberman has recently shown that such governance also undermines the effectiveness of the AIDS response:

> In ethnically divided societies, discources of risk were more likely to focus on particular ethnic groups than on the society at large, reducing the potential base of support for aggressive policies. The net effects were substantial in terms of expenditure levels, prevention and treatment coverage, and the timing of certain policies. Although more recent years have witnessed increasing convergence and coordination across countries in their actions on AIDS, lost time has cost lives and magnified the epidemic. (2009, p. 292)

The effectiveness of the response to AIDS has been undermined by the political logic of democratic governance in the African state.

The prospects for vertical accountability

Although the notion of 'accountable leadership' is central to democratic governance, neo-patrimonialism leads to the suppression of political competition and accountability in order to sustain one particular political elite through consecutive electoral cycles (van de Walle 2007). In such a system, political stakeholders that have formal powers to hold the executive to account are unlikely to do so as they are 'clients' whose positions and careers depend on their loyalty to the president. Such loyalties prevent the use of horizontal accountability between governance institutions, but the logic applies also vertically. Herbert Kitschelt and Steven Wilkinson argue that, in such political systems, the true nature of party-voter linkages is best captured by the notion of '*clientelistic accountability* [which] represents a transaction, the direct exchange of a citizen's vote in return for direct payments or continuing access to employment, goods and services' (2007, p. 2).

Our review of the literature would suggest that vertical accountability is an unlikely governance mechanism for leveraging more effective responses to AIDS. This conclusion has support in empirical research on data collected by the Afrobarometer. In explaining electoral choice, Michael Bratton and his colleagues find statistical support for both the cultural and evaluation hypotheses, and they identify how the influence of ethnic identity varies depending on the number and relative size of ethnic groups in the country (2005, pp. 304–308). The authors point out, however, that it would be a mistake to assume that voters' evaluations of government performance are always well-informed. On the contrary, the authors argue that:

> [T]he very absence of cognitive considerations in the formation of voting preferences points to the fact that election campaigns in African countries are conducted, if not in complete isolation from the truth, at least in environments where reliable information is hard to come by. (Bratton *et al.* 2005, pp. 307–308)

If evaluations of government performance are likely to be more or less misinformed, one would assume the risk for false evaluations to be particularly high on an issue such as the AIDS response that is difficult to evaluate as well as steeped in stigma and prejudice.

Finally, what can survey research tell us about voters' perceptions of elections? Do African voters see elections as opportunities to exert political pressure on poorly performing governments? On the basis of his research on Afrobarometer data, Robert Mattes concludes:

> Ordinary Africans demonstrate an incomplete grasp of political accountability. While they are willing to play a more questioning and critical role toward the state, they still hold paternalistic views of that state. They clearly support multi-party elections, and want their legislators to remain close at hand. But they appear to support elections as a mechanism of choice rather than as a means of controlling the behaviour of their representatives by threatening to withhold their vote. (Mattes 2010, p. 20)

The percentage of voters who see elections as opportunities to sanction politicians varies between African countries, with the nature of the electoral system being the strongest determinant. People in countries with large-list proportional representation systems – as in South Africa and Namibia – are less likely to view elections in that light. Other than this institutional factor, voters who hold the opinion that the government works for people are, quite naturally, more likely to see elections as an opportunity to fire the government.

This review of literature leads to the conclusion that, due to the nature of political governance and people's perceptions of elections, it is unlikely that public opinion on AIDS will be an incentive for government to provide stronger and more accountable leadership in the response to AIDS. This general conclusion does not deny that public opinion is one of several political resource that should be mobilised for the long-term realisation of essential targets in relation to AIDS, health and development. Such a mobilisation is more likely to succeed if we better understand some central features of public opinion on AIDS and what political factors and individual-level determinants shape that opinion.

Describing public opinion on AIDS

The public opinion data on HIV and AIDS will be presented and analysed in a few steps, starting with the presentation of frequencies and ending off with the results from a set of multivariate logistic regression analyses. The four rounds of the Afrobarometer surveys contain the same two questions that form the basis for this analysis. The first question is *In your opinion, what are the most important problems facing this country that government should address?* The respondent is asked to name three problems which are coded by the interviewer. The variable referred to as 'AIDS MIP' (Most Important Problem) in Table 1 is a dichotomous variable that distinguishes between the respondents who named HIV and AIDS as one of the three problems and those who did not. The second question is *How well or badly would you say the current government is [combating HIV/AIDS], or haven't you heard enough to say?* It is important to note that the respondent is not asked to give a reason for her evaluation of the government's performance. The third variable – 'AIDS constituency' – was computed by combining the first two variables so that it identifies the respondents who named HIV and AIDS as one of the three most important problems *and* who were critical of how the government handled the response to AIDS. These are the respondents who arguably would be more likely to allow their opinions about AIDS and the government's response to influence their electoral preference in the next election.

Table 1 lists the percentages of respondents in each country who hold the three opinions in each of the four rounds of the *Afrobarometer* surveys.

With the exception of Botswana, Namibia and South Africa, the percentage of people who prioritise AIDS on the public agenda is very low and decreasing. The regional average percentages of people who are critical of how their government has responded to AIDS are by far the highest of the three opinions. It is the majority opinion in South Africa and Zimbabwe in three of the surveys. The AIDS constituency, finally, is exceptionally small, with an average of only 1.2% in 2008. South Africa is the clear exception with an AIDS constituency 10 times larger than the regional average.

But are these opinions 'correct', in the sense that they reflect the severity of the epidemic and a level of effort by governments that can be assessed objectively, or are they more or less misinformed opinions that may shift for reasons that have little to do with the epidemic and the quality of the government's response? A thorough answer to that question lies beyond the scope of this paper. The ambition here is therefore limited to exploring correlations with relevant factors.

Linking opinion and objective data

An attempt to see if the nature of public opinion reflects the epidemic or the quality of the response is hampered by the fact that there is no generally accepted metric for assessing the level of effort by governments (Fox *et al*. 2011). The analysis will therefore rely on proxy indicators. The severity of the epidemic will be captured by HIV prevalence and the estimated number of AIDS-related deaths per 100,000 people, with data from UNAIDS (2010). We would expect both these variables to correlate positively with the number of people who think AIDS is one of the three most important problems, since the social effects of both higher prevalence and AIDS-related deaths would mobilise public opinion throughout society. We would expect those social effects to also generate a correlation with the level of criticism

Table 1. Public opinion on HIV and AIDS in Africa (% of national samples).

Country	1999/2001 AIDS MIP	1999/2001 Critical of government	1999/2001 AIDS constituency	2003/2004 AIDS MIP	2003/2004 Critical of government	2003/2004 AIDS constituency	2005/2006 AIDS MIP	2005/2006 Critical of government	2005/2006 AIDS constituency	2008 AIDS MIP	2008 Critical of government	2008 AIDS constituency
Benin	–	–	–	–	–	–	0.8	25.0	0.2	0.7	30.8	0.3
Botswana	20.1	0.0	0.0	29.1	21.3	4.8	27.1	7.0	1.4	10.8	4.8	0.6
Burkina Faso	–	–	–	–	–	–	–	–	–	0.5	19.8	0.2
Cape Verde	–	–	–	2.4	25.3	0.9	2.4	11.0	0.2	0.9	21.7	0.2
Ghana	–	–	–	3.1	12.5	0.7	0.5	12.8	0.1	0.8	15.1	0.0
Kenya	–	–	–	9.3	16.7	1.3	4.5	21.0	0.8	2.1	20.1	0.5
Lesotho	0.1	0.0	0.0	4.8	26.0	1.3	5.0	27.0	2.3	4.0	16.7	1.2
Liberia	–	–	–	–	–	–	–	–	–	0.3	27.3	0.1
Madagascar	–	–	–	–	–	–	0.3	8.4	0.1	0.4	11.0	0.1
Malawi	1.0	0.0	0.0	2.7	48.1	1.6	1.0	36.8	0.3	2.1	13.4	0.0
Mali	0.0	18.1	0.0	0.5	18.1	0.2	0.5	10.0	0.0	0.7	18.1	0.1
Mozambique	–	–	–	12.5	39.4	4.6	6.3	24.9	2.0	4.6	18.8	0.9
Namibia	10.7	0.0	0.0	28.0	33.0	11.6	23.2	27.7	8.3	9.6	26.1	4.4
Nigeria	–	–	–	3.7	29.4	1.2	1.8	40.9	0.8	2.0	34.9	0.9
Senegal	–	–	–	0.9	13.3	0.1	0.7	11.6	0.2	0.3	13.5	0.0
South Africa	7.9	56.8	5.3	26.8	47.4	14.8	23.9	40.5	10.4	20.5	56.5	12.1
Tanzania	0.4	26.5	0.0	13.6	20.4	3.0	3.3	13.0	0.6	3.4	14.8	0.9
Uganda	0.4	21.6	0.2	7.2	22.7	2.4	6.0	13.4	0.9	4.6	26.4	1.3
Zambia	–	–	–	3.2	31.4	1.2	5.6	22.3	1.6	1.2	22.2	0.4
Zimbabwe	3.3	0.0	0.0	6.5	28.8	2.4	7.8	59.7	5.1	0.4	23.0	0.1
Average	4.9	13.7	0.6	9.6	27.1	3.3	6.7	22.9	2.0	3.5	21.7	1.2

Notes: Three public opinions on AIDS in Africa. The last row gives the average percentages.
Source: Afrobarometer public opinion surveys, rounds 1–4. The notation '–' implies that the country was not included in that round of the survey.

of the government's response, but since Table 1 shows that there are high levels of criticism also in countries with relatively low levels of prevalence, no such correlation should be expected.

The proxy indicators for government effort in the response is the coverage percentage of antiretroviral medication (ARV), a very tangible effort that government can take some credit for. While people may understand that the level of coverage also depends on efforts by non-governmental actors, it is nevertheless likely that opinions of the government effort are less critical in countries with a high ARV coverage – a negative correlation. The results of the analyses can be found in Table 2.

The results confirm the reasoning above, with one exception. The correlation is strong and positive between, on the one hand, HIV prevalence and AIDS mortality and, on the other, the variable AIDS MIP. As a consequence of how it was constructed, a similar but somewhat weaker links exist to the variable AIDS constituency. As expected, there is no correlation with the percentage of people who are critical of government efforts.

The more surprising result is that governments are not rewarded for the coverage of ARVs, an effort that varies between 4% for Madagascar and 95% for Namibia and Botswana. Even though the correlation is negative, as expected, it is weak and not statistically significant. The lack of traction between these two variables can be given several alternative interpretations, of which the most likely, arguably, is that people in general are just not aware of the coverage statistics and can therefore not consider it when shaping their opinion of the government's effort. In this regard, Botswana appear to be the clear exception with decreasing levels of criticism as the country has reached virtually full ARV coverage. The severity of the HIV epidemic in the societies is a more common awareness that generates criticism also in countries where the epidemic is less severe in a regional comparison. We can conclude that since the level of criticism of government is relatively high across all countries, the variation in the size of the AIDS constituency depends on the extent to which people prioritise HIV and AIDS as an issue that government should address.

Further insights can be gained by visualising the correlation between HIV prevalence and the variable AIDS MIP, see Figure 1.

On the lower end of the prevalence scale, up until 10–12%, the countries are all close to the regression line – the 'model' that is superimposed on the countries – but there is much greater variation among the countries with the most severe epidemics. An interpretation that would be consistent with this data would be to say that, given the many other problems faced by the people in the region, HIV and AIDS is a central issue in the public discourse only in the countries with the most severe epidemics. At that level of impact, the degree to which the public thinks HIV and AIDS is one of the most important problems depends on the degree to which there is political space in civil society and a free media to mobilise support for such an argument. The key

Table 2. Correlating aggregate public opinion to objective data, 2008/2009.

	HIV prevalence	AIDS mortality	ARV coverage
AIDS MIP	0.723**	0.597**	0.267
Critical of government	0.110	0.154	−0.090
AIDS constituency	0.565*	495*	0.166

Note: Correlation coefficients (Pearson's r) between the three opinion variables in Table 1 and HIV prevalence, the number of estimated AIDS-related deaths per 100,000 people, and the percentage of coverage of ARV treatment. Source: Afrobarometer (round 4) and UNAIDS (2010).
*$p < 0.05$.
**$p < 0.01$.
$N = 20$.

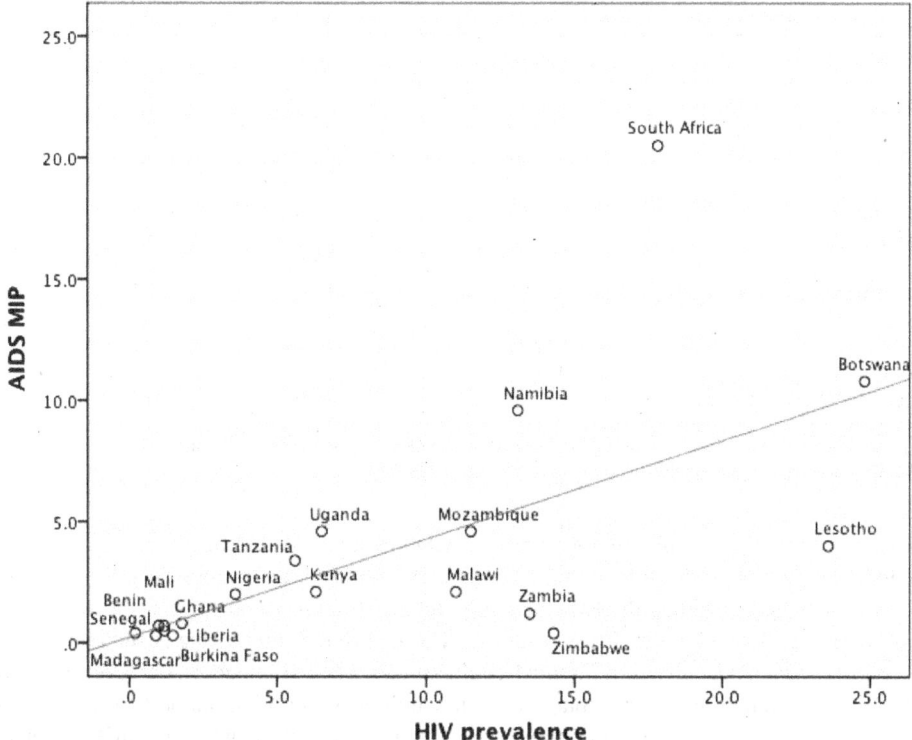

Figure 1. Visualising the link between HIV prevalence and public opinion. The figure shows the scatter plot graph of the two variables HIV prevalence (2009) and AIDS MIP, as explained in the text.
Source: UNAIDS (2010) and Afrobarometer public opinion survey round 4.

here is to remember that the Afrobarometer question is not just whether AIDS is a serious threat to society, but whether it is a questions that the *government must address*. At roughly the same level of impact from AIDS, the main difference in the opinions on AIDS between people in South Africa and people in Zambia, Zimbabwe and Lesotho, is not necessarily their understanding of the severity of the threat, but whether it is understood to be a problem that should be addressed in the public political realm or at the level of personal morality.

The nature of AIDS constituencies

The last section of the paper will explore the construct 'AIDS constituency' in some further detail. How does this constituency compare with constituencies for other issues, and can we identify any determinants of membership in the AIDS constituency that may suggest strategies to boost its size in the interest of leveraging a stronger AIDS response?

When the full Afrobarometer sample is considered, the five most common problems that respondents feel their government should address are unemployment, poverty, food shortage, health and education. The size of the constituencies for three of these issues, together with the AIDS constituency, are listed in Table 3 for the 11 countries with the most severe epidemics.

It is not surprising that unemployment and poverty top the list as the biggest issue constituencies as they both capture concerns directly relating to economic prospects for a better future. In the research by Bratton that was cited above, these are the issues that voters base their evaluation of performance upon. The dominance of these two issues also reflect the findings

Table 3. Comparing issue constituencies.

	Unemployment	Poverty	Health	AIDS
Botswana	45.7	16.1	3.4	0.6
Kenya	27.4	20.4	5.9	0.5
Lesotho	42.8	20.3	3.8	1.2
Malawi	5.3	10.0	5.4	0.0
Mozambique	21.2	9.8	6.8	0.9
Namibia	36.3	19.0	4.5	4.4
Nigeria	37.5	24.6	5.7	0.9
South Africa	39.5	12.8	7.7	12.1
Uganda	21.8	32.2	13.0	1.3
Zambia	26.7	24.6	27.8	0.4
Zimbabwe	16.4	6.2	9.7	0.1
Average for all 20 countries	25.5	16.9	10.7	1.2

Note: Percentages of respondents belonging to 'issue constituencies' in a selection of countries.
Source: Afrobarometer public opinion survey, round 4 from 2008/2009.

by Justesen (2011) that people do not prioritise AIDS as a political issues because of their very immediate struggles to survive in a context of poverty. Of more direct relevance to this paper is the size of the poverty and health constituencies, and the strategic opportunities this may suggest to boost demands for a stronger AIDS response. The fact that South Africa is such an outlier in the correlation that is visualised in Figure 1 could arguably be explained by the level of political and media freedom in South Africa that allows stakeholders to mobilise support for the argument that the AIDS response belong in the political realm and that is it the government's responsibility. But what strategies stakeholders use to put that message across would also matter. The fact that the AIDS constituency in South Africa is larger than the health constituency and roughly on par with the poverty constituency is probably a reflection of the success that the Treatment Action Campaign and some other civil society organisations has had with their strategy to link HIV and AIDS to broader concerns around poverty and health (Geffen 2010). South Africans who name AIDS as one of the most important issues are likely to do so knowing that an effective response would also address related health issues and combat poverty.

Knowing the individual-level determinants for belonging in the AIDS constituency might suggest further ways to boost the political leverage of public opinion on AIDS. In order to identify such characteristics, a set of multivariate logistic regression analyses were conducted with the dichotomous 'AIDS constituency' as the dependent variable. The explanatory variables in the analysis all refer back to four of the five competing explanations that were used in the analysis by Bratton, i.e. structural, cultural, institutional and cognitive characteristics. The one additional variable captures whether or not the respondent has lost a relative or a close friend to AIDS in order to test if there is a political effect from such personal loss.

In the full sample of 27,713 respondents in the fourth round of the Afrobarometer survey, only 459 individuals belong to the AIDS constituency. Since 291 of these respondents are South Africans, the same regression model was used first on the full regional sample and then again separately on the South African sub-sample as a way of distinguishing effects that were specific to the South African constituency. Further exploration of this data through more specified and country-specific analyses would yield additional and more nuanced information. The results of these initial explorations are detailed in Table 4.

The analysis that included all 20 countries show that members of the AIDS constituency have greater cognitive awareness, in terms of having higher levels of education and accessing more news reporting in the media, both of which would make them more able to assess the

Table 4. Determinants for inclusion in the AIDS constituency.

Independent variables	Regression coefficient (B), all countries	Regression coefficient (B), South Africa
Education	0.286**	–
News media consumption	0.432**	–
Political engagement	−0.098**	–
Active member in civil society organisation	−0.371**	–
Loyal to political party	0.391**	–
Importance of religion	−0.456**	−0.192**
Personal loss to AIDS	0.560**	0.754**
Citizen empowerment	–	0.193**
Model fit (Nagelkerke R^2)	0.073	0.042

Notes: Regression coefficients for the statistically significant determinants for inclusion in the AIDS constituency, for all countries and for South Africa, respectively. Data from Afrobarometer round 4.
**$p < 0.01$.

importance of AIDS and the quality of the government's response. Whereas members of the constituency are likely to identify with a political party, they are less likely to actively engage on political issues either informally or as members of civil society organisations. In terms of value systems, those with a religious frame of reference are far less likely to be part of the AIDS constituency. Irrespective of other differences, members of the AIDS constituency are likely to have had their opinions shaped by the experience of losing a friend or relative to AIDS. In combination, these characteristics conjure up the image of a relatively well-educated and politically aware African whose views are not dictated by any formal political attachments or religious prescriptions, a citizen whose opinions on the issue were triggered by the AIDS-related death of a loved one.

The analysis of the South African sub-sample gives us less to go on, as only three of the variables are statistically significant. As in the full sample, a religious outlook on life makes inclusion in the constituency less likely, and the experience of personal loss much more so. Members of the South African constituency, however, are also more likely to hold the view that government works for the citizens. This is the same perception of citizen empowerment that Robert Mattes identified as a determinant for using the vote as a means to effect vertical accountability.

On a more speculative note one could interpret these results to suggest that people are more likely to belong to the AIDS constituency when they realise that their own experience of personal loss to AIDS, and those of far too many others, can and should be traced back to a political failure to provide an effective response. In the region, such a realisation is more likely among people who are better educated and generally more informed of social and political dynamics, and who are free to shape their own opinions. In South Africa, where AIDS activists successfully have made this argument for some time now, this is understood by people irrespective of their educational background.

Conclusions

Against the backdrop of increasingly clear normative prescriptions for the AIDS response to be based on democratic governance principles in general and accountability in particular, this research set out to assess whether vertical accountability might provide effective leverage for a strong AIDS response in the region that needs it most – sub-Saharan Africa. One clear result of the analysis, which supports the findings in previous research, is that such leverage is unlikely to materialise across the region even in the medium term. In order for this to happen, one would need to see not only a drastic increase and shift in public awareness on AIDS, but also fundamental improvements in the quality of political governance in order for such opinions to shape political outcomes. Although there are country variations, there is arguably no general trend in the region towards such governance reforms, which means that any expectations on vertical accountability to make a difference in the quality of the AIDS response will remain frustrated.

This conclusion should not, however, be understood to suggest that stakeholders should give up on efforts to communicate with and try to shape the perceptions of the general public. Even if one should not expect results in the short or even mid-term, it is essential for the long-term sustainability of the AIDS response that it is supported by a politically relevant constituency in the general public. The campaign strategies that have been applied in South Africa might suggest avenues for how to frame issues differently in order to achieve greater political traction. The opportunity to tag such AIDS messaging onto efforts to reach the Millennium Development Goals by 2015 should not be underestimated.

In the absence of a large constituency that is supportive of an AIDS response that is effective also in terms of HIV prevention, the response will suffer a democratic deficit that presents an intricate governance dilemma. Incentive structures are currently not aligned to generate the necessary political opportunities and electoral rewards that would sustain accountable leadership in an effective response. The political reforms that would be necessary to ensure an effective response would greatly benefit development efforts far beyond the fight against HIV and AIDS. Better governance of the AIDS response would imply higher quality democratic governance more generally. The ambition should be no less.

Acknowledgements

The author is grateful to Sida and Norad for providing funding for this research through the Swedish/Norwegian HIV/AIDS team in Lusaka.

Note

1. The Afrobarometer project conducts nationally representative public opinion surveys on political, economic and social issues across sub-Saharan Africa. The interviews are conducted in local languages. For further information, see www.afrobarometer.org.

References

Bor, J., 2007. The political economy of AIDS leadership in developing countries: an exploratory analysis. *Social Science & Medicine*, 64 (8), 1585–1599.

Bratton, M., Mattes, R., and Gyimah-Boadi, E., 2005. *Public opinion, democracy and market reform in Africa*. Cambridge: Cambridge University Press.

Bratton, M., Bhavnani, R., and Chen, T.H., 2011. *Voting intensions in Africa: ethnic, economic or partisan?* Afrobarometer Working Paper No. 127, January 2011. Available from: www.afrobarometer.org [accessed 10 April 2012].

Diamond, L. and Morlino, L., 2005. Introduction. *In*: L. Diamond and L. Morlino, eds. *Assessing the quality of democracy*. Baltimore, MD: The Johns Hopkins University Press, ix–xliii.

Fox, A.M., *et al.*, 2011. Conceptual and methodological challenges to measuring political commitment to respond to HIV. *Journal of the International AIDS Society*, 14 (Suppl. 2), S5.

Geffen, N., 2010. *Debunking delusions: the inside story of the treatment action campaign*. Johannesburg: Jacana.

Hyden, G., 2006. *African politics in comparative perspective*. Cambridge: Cambridge University Press.

Irurzun-Lopez, M. and Poku, N., 2005. Pursuing African AIDS governance: consolidating the response and preparing for the future. *In*: A.S. Patterson, ed. *The African state and the AIDS crisis*. London: Ashgate, 219–230.

Justesen, M.K., 2011. *Too poor to care? The salience of AIDS in Africa*. Afrobarometer Working Paper No. 133. Available from: www.afrobarometer.org [accessed 10 April 2012].

Kitschelt, H. and Wilkinson, S.I., 2007. Citizen-politician linkages: an introduction. *In*: H. Kitschelt and S.I. Wilkinson, eds. *Patrons, clients, and policies: patterns of democratic accountability and political competition*. Cambridge: Cambridge University Press, 1–49.

Lieberman, E.S., 2009. *Boundaries of contagion: how ethnic politics have shaped government responses to HIV/AIDS*. Princeton, NJ: Princeton University Press.

Mattes, R., 2004. *Public opinion on AIDS: facing up to the future?* Afrobarometer briefing paper, no. 12 (April 2004). Available from: www.afrobarometer.org [accessed 10 April 2012].

Mattes, R., 2010. Controlling power – African's views on governance, citizenship and accountability. *In*: M. Claase and C. Alpin-Lardies, eds. *Social accountability in Africa: practitioners' experiences and lessons*. Cape Town: IDASA, 8–22.

Poku, N.K., 2005. *AIDS in Africa: how the poor are dying*. Cambridge: Polity Press.

Posner, D.N., 2006. *Institutions and ethnic politics in Africa*. Cambridge: Cambridge University Press.

Schmitter, P., 2005. The ambiguous virtues of accountability. *In*: L. Diamond and L. Morlino, eds. *Assessing the Quality of Democracy*. Baltimore, MD: The Johns Hopkins University Press, 18–31.

Strand, P., Kinney, M., and Mattes, R., 2008. Politics and policy outcomes on children affected by HIV/AIDS in Africa. *IDS Bulletin*, 39 (5), 80–87.

UNAIDS, 2010. *Global report: UNAIDS report on the global AIDS epidemic*. Geneva: UNAIDS.

United Nations, 2011. *Political declaration on HIV/AIDS: intensifying our efforts to eliminate HIV/AIDS*. UN General Assembly Resolution 65/277, adopted 10 June 2011.

van de Walle, N., 2007. Meet the new boss, same as the old boss? The evolution of political clientelism in Africa. *In*: H. Kitschelt and S.I. Wilkinson, eds. *Patrons, clients, and policies: patterns of democratic accountability and political competition*. Cambridge: Cambridge University Press, 50–67.

de Waal, A., 2006. *AIDS and power: why there is no political crisis – yet*. London: Zed Books.

Whiteside, A., Mattes, R., Willan, S., and Manning, R., 2004. What people really believe about HIV/AIDS in Southern Africa. *In*: N.K. Poku and A. Whiteside, eds. *The political economy of AIDS in Africa*. London: Ashgate, 127–149.

Whiteside, A., 2007. HIV/AIDS and development: failures of vision and imagination. *In*: N. Poku, A. Whiteside and B. Sandkjaer, eds. *AIDS and governance*. London: Ashgate, 115–131.

Building capacities and producing citizens: the biopolitics of HIV prevention in Brazil

Rafael de la Dehesa and Ananya Mukherjea

Capacity-building has become a mainstay of many AIDS and public health programmes. This article examines its impact on civil society organisations and claims-making around citizenship, as these have been articulated through heterogeneous policy networks doing HIV prevention work. Drawing on a growing literature on the Foucauldian notions of biopower and governmentality, the genealogy of capacity-building as a globalised technology of governmentality is traced, examining its uses both at the international level and in Brazil. Brazilian civil society organisations have undoubtedly been transformed by their participation in networks carrying out capacity-building projects. While recognising these effects, the conflicts and productive tensions inherent to such networks are highlighted.

In 2004, the Joint United Nations programme on HIV/AIDS and the Brazilian government announced the creation of the International Centre for Technical Cooperation on HIV/AIDS within the Brazilian National STD/AIDS programme. With the goal of '[strengthening] the capacities' of developing countries' response to the epidemic, the new centre would facilitate 'South–South' technical cooperation, drawing on the experience of multiple actors. Within three years, it had attracted funds from various international agencies and built a network of 74 primarily nongovernmental organisations (NGOs) from Brazil and elsewhere but also state agencies to work on projects in the areas of advocacy, strengthening civil society, and prevention among 'vulnerable populations', again with an important emphasis on capacity-building (CICT 2008). At one level, the initiative could be read against a shifting geopolitical landscape in which Brazil has played an increasingly prominent role, as an effort to capitalise on the much-touted 'Brazilian response' to the epidemic. Through measures combining broad-based prevention efforts, the extensive incorporation of civil society organisations, and universal access to medicines, Brazil has succeeded in halving the number of HIV cases predicted a decade ago and sharply reducing the number of deaths (Biehl 2004). Yet, in its articulation of multiple actors, particularly in the prominent role played by NGOs, and in its ambition to mobilise diffuse capacities latent in societies, the initiative also reflects emerging frameworks of management that are decentring (though not displacing) the nation-state, to some extent recasting the parameters of citizenship, and that speak to the emergence of HIV at a time of neoliberal ascendance.

The AIDS epidemic has been primary among many global forces in fostering the incorporation of civil society into the formulation and implementation of policy, both internationally and, in many countries, nationally. In this respect, HIV/AIDS policy is but one expression of broader transformations unfolding in the current context of globalisation. To understand the impact of these changes on civil society and claims-making around citizenship in the response to the epidemic, we draw on Foucault's notions of governmentality and biopower. Governmentality, broadly, refers to political rationalities and administrative techniques designed to manage individual and collective conduct towards the realisation of collective wellbeing. Governmentality is associated historically with the emergence of biopower, a modern form of governance that brought life processes (fertility, mortality, morbidity, etc.) into the purview of rationalised administration.[1]

Neoliberal governing technologies, grounded in notions of corporate organisation and market calculations, represent merely the most recent of these techniques to administer life. Their hallmarks include an organisational reliance on policy networks, flexible and heterogeneous arrangements that may include national and transnational, state and non-state actors engaged in the exchange of information and resources and in coordinated efforts around the formulation and implementation of policy (Chalmers *et al.* 1997, Keck and Sikkink 1998, Torres-Ruiz 2011).[2] Such networks, in turn, often rely on the subjectification of clearly bounded populations, seeking to induce their self-government through a kind of 'regulatory enframing' designed to optimise choices, as in the adoption of safe-sex practices (Burchell 1996, Ong 2006). As Foucault (2008, p. 259) suggested in *The Birth of Biopolitics*, neoliberal governmentality marks a partial move away from an 'exhaustively disciplinary society', with its central distinction between normalised populations and those who cannot be normalised and are therefore excluded and towards a society organised around the 'optimization of systems of difference ... in which minority individuals and practices are tolerated'. The optimal sex worker, for instance, is the one who understands prevention, can negotiate safe sex, and exerts active agency in her social environment. This gradual shift towards optimisation, of course, creates its own barriers and invisibilities. However, while numerous populations subsist beyond the boundaries of citizenship or the possibility for citizenship, NGOs' emerging role in governance has also allowed some groups that would once have been similarly marginalised to find new legitimacy in advancing rights-based claims.

Against this backdrop of evolving technologies of governmentality, capacity-building has become a mainstay of many public health and HIV/AIDS programmes. The Declaration of Commitment reached at the UN General Assembly's Special Session on HIV/AIDS in 2001, for instance, calls for strengthening the capacities of: health, education, and legal systems; women and adolescent girls; governments, families, and communities; national research facilities and labs; and developing countries in general. Yet, the language of 'capacity-building' can be euphemistic or obscure, as when used to indicate certain 'citizen-like' behaviours. We understand capacity-building to encompass an array of goals, expectations, and policy prescriptions aimed at both organisations and ordinary citizens, which may include: (1) the transmission of knowledge and skills; (2) the validation of local and experiential knowledge and its incorporation into policy; (3) the production of infrastructure and organisational capacities (mission statements, project proposals, etc.); and (4) the promotion of specific types of subjectivity through deeper 'practices of self', in Foucauldian terms, as in workshops that promote self-esteem as a conduit for AIDS prevention. While we recognise that all these elements may fall under the rubric of 'capacity-building', our interest in this question is partly informed by the fact those engaged with it may hold conflicting expectations. As the concept has become ubiquitous and more mutable in its meanings, attention to its political implications is increasingly necessary.

In this article, we focus specifically on capacity-building efforts involving civil society organisations because of their implications for social movements and claims-making around citizenship. While we do not explore capacity-building targeting other actors participating in the response to the epidemic (clinical laboratories; healthcare providers; government agencies, etc.), the coexistence of all these efforts underscores its reliance on heterogeneous actors, often articulated through policy networks. Drawing on a growing literature on biopower and governmentality (Foucault 1991, 2008, Burchell 1996, Cruikshank 1996, Biehl 2004, Ong 2006), we trace the genealogy of capacity-building as a globalised technology of governmentality particularly salient in HIV/AIDS prevention, examining its uses both at the international level and in Brazil. We consider Brazil in particular because its response to the epidemic has been broadly touted as a model for the Global South and because it has undertaken internationally recognised measures to incorporate capacity-building into HIV/AIDS prevention. In examining capacity-building as a technology at once national and transnational, we suggest that competing interests among those involved belie understandings of governmentality as a seamless web of biopolitical management. In Brazil, networks administering capacity-building projects have undoubtedly transformed civil society organisations. We recognise this, but we also highlight the tensions and potential conflicts inherent to such networks, which in Brazil, have expanded the purview of both HIV/AIDS prevention and claims-making around citizenship. This article is based largely on documents produced by international agencies as well as the National programme and activist organisations in Brazil, though it is also informed by a larger research project that involved over 100 interviews with primarily lesbian, gay, bisexual, and transgender (LGBT) but also sex worker and AIDS activists as well as National programme officials (De la Dehesa 2010).

Vulnerability, networks, and capacity-building

Chambre (2006, p. xi) writes that '... the AIDS community [in New York in the early 1980s] formed to respond to a complex medical condition and to the limitations of the contemporary healthcare system'. HIV/AIDS organising was essential for those most vulnerable to the disease and its effects, providing oversight for the municipal healthcare system and supplementing its services with more useful ones. This coalescence of a group of suffering and at-risk individuals to address the common cause of reducing the rate of HIV infections and AIDS-related deaths was as unexpected as it was ultimately essential amidst the panic and confusion surrounding the emergence of AIDS in the USA as in many other countries. That such networks of agents invested in the pandemic have continued to grow (and to form a looser if larger global mesh of networks) as the disease has become increasingly settled into poor and disenfranchised populations continues to be socially and politically remarkable 30 years later. Governments and healthcare providers have come to rely on them for the production and dissemination of information and as sources of volunteers, advisers, workers, and observers. Changing the face of HIV prevention, AIDS care, and knowledge production about the disease, they have also become a model of how activists can affect policy (Altman 1994, Torres-Ruiz 2011). Yet, the structured relations within and among networks necessarily raise questions about governance and representation.

Networks range from purely social, interpersonal connexions to highly formalised contractual arrangements that might encompass NGOs, government agencies, research centres, corporations, funders, and international agencies. The growing salience of networks as a technique of governmentality speaks to the neoliberal decentring of the state, with NGOs and other actors coming to play a compensatory role at the limits of state action (Chalmers *et al.* 1997). As sociologists Chambre (2006) and Epstein (1996) describe their development, networks may form around a shared identity or common cause emerging from a perceived shared vulnerability, creating 'a sense of common interest in achieving particular goals' (Campbell 2003, p. 59). This perception may be internal to their membership, as was the case with gay men in the USA in the early 1980s whose friends and lovers were becoming ill, or external. Indeed, even more organically formed networks can alter their membership, presentation, or priorities to meet the expectations of governments, funders, or international agencies.

Alliances grounded in the perception of shared vulnerabilities are central to networks' governance and governing functions. As Treichler (1999, p. 235) observes, 'An effective response to an epidemic ... depends on the existence of identities *for whom that epidemic is meaningful* – and stories in which *those identities are taken up and animated*' (emphasis ours). Identities (sex worker, *travesti*, homeless, etc.) are thus reified and made deployable though also strategically altered as networks dynamically evolve. Framing the best possible responses to conditions of vulnerability, these points of alliance are optimised into figures both informed and representative though, sometimes, less representative of all members of the 'target population' over time. Guta *et al.* (2011) describe the 'professionalization' of peer-advocate-clients at community-based organisations offering harm reduction services, who must learn to behave like upper-level workers, for instance, participating in long meetings despite experiencing severe heroin withdrawal symptoms. Tasked with explicitly representing marginalised populations (injection drug users; the chronically unemployed), they must implicitly behave like more formalised workers. Similarly, as the popular image of the risky bisexual man of early AIDS panics in the USA slowly morphed into that of the safer-sex-practising, HIV-knowledgeable gay man, associated stigmas were countered by notions of many gay men as expert-activists (Epstein 1996), even as other at-risk men who have sex with men slipped into obscurity, beyond the reach of most prevention and treatment programmes. Patton (1990), among others, has underscored the slippage that occurs between the populations identified as in need or most vulnerable and the individuals who come to represent, or liaise with, those needs. To the extent that identity categories or points of affiliation become sedimented in public policy, such slippage is inherent to biopolitical practices (Ong 2006).

Writing of the South African Treatment Action Campaign, Grebe (2008) suggests that policy networks are dynamic coalitions of agents who rely on a sometimes tense and delicate balance of interpersonal trust, which often precedes the formation of the group, and on complementary skills and interests. Political scientists Keck and Sikkink (1998, pp. 89–90) point out that networks are 'communicative structures', where activists seek 'not only to influence policy outcomes, but to transform the terms and nature of the debate'. They are, therefore, ultimately, *systems of negotiation* about resources, knowledge production, status, political, and social goals, as well as the structures of governance, both internal to a network and with outside organisations.

The promotion of community responses to HIV/AIDS requires the utilisation of civil society networks as communicative structures and instruments of policy implementation and programme development. towards these goals, the policy network also functions as a mediator of capacities within communities. For example, the peers in the South African township about which Campbell (2003, p. 59) writes demanded structural responses to the immediate physical violence in their daily lives. When authorities within the township instead threatened physical violence to persuade the peers to continue their work without change, prevention efforts stalled and sputtered.

Agencies interested in capacity-building often foster the consolidation of organic networks into more highly structured groups. In the 1990s, for example, India's national government routed funds from the World Bank to local public health programmers in West Bengal, and they produced a multi-stakeholders format for the ultimately effective HIV prevention project in red light districts there (Jana *et al.* 2004). The successes of this programme over the following decade contributed to the production of a complex system of capacity-building mechanisms for local sex workers – male, female, and transgender, with or without formal immigrant or citizen status – as well as their clients. These capacity-building mechanisms comprised literacy training, legal workshops, and grooming sex workers to appear at public forums. The sex workers formed strong labour unions, though such representation was sometimes nominal or incomplete. The question of the most liminal of sex workers (the very young, the forcibly trafficked) remains fraught, but individual organisers and their constituencies did achieve boosted status and visibility through the formation of such a policy network.

Policy networks have been central to and influential in the development of responses to HIV/AIDS since its inception, as a means of organising populations around the concept of shared vulnerability, fostering alliances within and across groups, and mobilising systems of power-knowledge in technologies of government. However, in the definition and redefinition of network borders, some of the most liminal members of those populations have been excluded, left to a nebulous status outside citizenship. Moreover, while sometimes imagined as idealised expressions of horizontality and democratic deliberation, networks are not free of power asymmetries, which condition both access to them and dynamics among NGOs of varying capacities and between NGOs and state and international bodies, particularly funders (Chalmers *et al.* 1997). Shared or overlapping capacity-building goals often comprise the meeting point around which actors can coalesce.

The concept of 'capacity building' has become a constant in the discourse of development. Derived from the post-Bretton-Woods notion of 'institution building', establishing the structures necessary to develop economies in debtor nations, capacity-building arrived in its present form at the UN Conference on Environment and Development, held in Rio de Janeiro in 1992. Chapter 37 of Agenda 21, produced at the meeting, titled, 'Creating capacity for sustainable development', states:

> A country's ability to develop more sustainably depends on the capacity of its people and institutions to understand complex environment and development issues so that they can make the right development choices... A fundamental goal of capacity building is to enhance the ability to evaluate and address the crucial questions related to policy choices and modes of implementation amongst development options, based on an understanding of environment potentials and limits and of *needs perceived by the people of the country concerned.* (Emphasis added)[3]

The shift in focus from restructuring debtor nations to providing support for their sustainable development is a hallmark of the new language. Questions relating to governmentality – of agency, the circulation of power, and the agendas being served – remain. Supporters of the language or principles of capacity development argue that the concept grants a formal place at the table to those 'stakeholders', like community-based activists or labourers in underground economies, who would previously only have been acted upon rather than involved in the process. Critics of the concept counter that only the name has changed and that the bulk of capacity development ultimately aims to further a neoliberal agenda and ensure the expansion of and compliance with trade agreements (George 2004).

As capacity-building has become a mainstay of many public health and HIV/AIDS programmes, it has become necessary for organisations to prioritise this in order to garner grant money. Through that process, the multiple meanings of the term can become confusing, as when it is used to indicate certain 'citizen-like' behaviours as a prerequisite for employment with an organisation or to refer to an individual's representative position on a grant application ('So-and-so, who is HIV+, will be doing capacity-building with others in her/his community').

This confusion in part reflects the concept's multi-stranded genealogy. As Altman (1994, p. 18) has suggested, the new global interest in community organising stemmed *both* from a commitment to grassroots participation and from an interest in rolling back the state, leading to 'sometimes strange alliances ... between new right and new left critiques of the state'. Eade (1997), in enumerating what capacity-building is *not*, specifies that it should not create dependency, should not weaken the state, and should not be pursued separate from other health and education programmes. Crucially, Eade points out that capacity-building is not synonymous with financial self-reliance and that some critical activities – such as the provision of healthcare and education – will always rely on robust funding, from international sources if necessary.

Both Farmer and Eade, in implicitly and explicitly invoke the tenets of liberation theology to support more humane, close-to-the-ground, and directly effective social justice goals. Eade specifies, 'Overall, a capacity-building approach is more concerned with enhancing people's capacity to articulate their own interests than with strengthening institutions *per se*'. And, in *Pathologies of Power*, Farmer (2004, p. 144) suggests that the goals of public health and development must be determined by existing needs and that admitting market forces or economic prescriptions to discipline debtor nations as significant factors, far from building real capacities, would constitute a human rights abuse. Farmer presents the simple idea that development and aid mechanisms should serve *needs* rather than markets and that needs and priorities should be determined largely by those citizens with the most at stake. While this philosophical dimension of Brazil's national response has served as an international model, the contradictions embedded in the concept's complex evolution and institutional expression through policy networks are evident.

Capacity-building and the Brazilian response

Appreciating the history of the AIDS movement in Brazil requires understanding the broader political landscape in which it emerged, one marked by the mass mobilisation ushered in by *abertura*, the gradual democratic opening announced by the military government (1964–1985) in the late 1970s. This larger context of contestation gave rise to a progressive healthcare reform movement that would play a critical role in the course of policy. Against narrowly epidemiological approaches to public health, this movement advanced a solidaristic vision of 'collective health' that underscored the societal dimensions of illness, understanding healthcare as a basic social right requiring the incorporation of excluded groups. The movement successfully pressed for the recognition of the right to healthcare in the 1988 constitution and for the creation of the country's Universal Healthcare System (SUS) based on principles of public sector responsibility, universal access, decentralised administration, and civic participation (Petchesky 2003). According to the political scientist Fleury (1997, pp. 28–36), an important participant in the movement, as healthcare reformers sought to translate their political beliefs into institutional arrangements, they saw decentralisation as a mechanism that could ensure greater 'societal control and political participation'. Given the power of local political machines in many areas, however, reformers envisioned arrangements of 'co-management' that could 'alter the bases of local power', albeit in ways that 'contradicted representative democracy by creating sectoral mechanisms of representation linked directly to the Executive'. To this end, popular healthcare councils were created at the local, state, and national levels that required representation by civil society organisations with the goal of making SUS more transparent and permeable to societal demands.

This broader push to democratise healthcare would shape both the Brazilian AIDS movement and the political terrain it encountered. As was the case in a number of other countries, civil society initiated the first organised responses to HIV. A homosexual liberation movement had emerged in the country in 1978, and after the first cases of AIDS were reported in the early 1980s, gay groups like the Grupo Gay da Bahia in Salvador began distributing pamphlets with the little information available on the disease. The establishment of the AIDS Prevention and Support Group (GAPA) in Sao Paulo in 1985 and the Brazilian Interdisciplinary AIDS Association (ABIA) in Rio de Janeiro the following year marked the emergence of an autonomous AIDS movement. Like other NGOs, a new phenomenon in the 1980s, AIDS NGOs had roots in the broader democratic opposition but distinguished themselves from other social movement organisations by their base among urban intellectuals, their professionalisation, their role as purveyors of specialised knowledge, and their ties to international foundations (Câmara da Silva 1998, Ramos 2004). The healthcare reform movement's influence on AIDS activism found expression ideologically, in its emphasis on principles of solidarity, social inclusion, and civic participation, and organisationally, in the importance of deliberative spaces like the National Meetings of AIDS NGOs (ENONGs), held annually and then biannually since 1989, where activists reach resolutions on the course of AIDS policy and elect representatives to the National AIDS Commission and other public bodies (Granjeiro et al. 2009).

The first state response to the epidemic not only in Brazil but in Latin America was the AIDS Reference and Treatment Centre established in the state of São Paulo in 1983. In 1985, the federal government issued guidelines for the creation of the National STD/AIDS programme, which began operating the following year. For several years, relations between the National programme and the AIDS movement remained fairly contentious, as activists decried the weakness and narrow biomedical focus of the government response. The notion of 'civil death', introduced by long-time leftist militant and AIDS activist Herbert Daniel, directly challenged the government neglect that inscribed people living with HIV/AIDS outside the realm of citizenship and public policy, leaving them to die. 'To affirm myself as a citizen who is perfectly alive is an act of civil disobedience', wrote Daniel (1994, p. 39) reflecting a politics of vitality that characterised much of civil society's response during the first decade of the epidemic. As sociologist Cristina Câmara da Silva (1998, p. 136) observes, such a politics sought to 'insert [people living with HIV/AIDS] into collective life and to displace individualised guilt and victimization onto the process of social relations'. Activists' relations with the government reached a low point during the administration of President Fernando Collor (1990–1992), when, against a backdrop of economic crisis and political instability, programme operations ground to a halt. These dynamics began to change in 1992, when the programme created an NGO Articulation Unit in the context of negotiations for the first of a series of World Bank loans. The first major experiment in capacity-building, however, began prior to the Bank's involvement.[4]

In 1989, the National programme launched Previna, a prevention project targeting 'high-risk groups', initially identified as prostitutes, intravenous drug users, and incarcerated populations, though subsequently expanded to other groups, including MSMs (Davida 1998). While limited in scope, Previna established several precedents for the organisation of subsequent capacity-building projects. As the programme's first major experiment in public–private partnerships with NGOs, oversight committees were established for each target population, incorporating activists and state officials, with the objective of producing educational materials for state and municipal workers on the targeted populations' medical needs and materials on prevention to be distributed with male condoms by peer educators, or *multiplicadores* ('multiplying agents'), among the populations themselves (Campos 2005). In the case of female sex workers, for example, the first organisational meeting brought together National programme officials, coordinators of STD/AIDS programmes from three states, and representatives of AIDS NGOs and sex worker organisations, including a French NGO working with sex workers in the state of Ceará (Ministerio da Saúde 2002). Officials also contracted the Prostitution and Human Rights programme of the Institute of Religious Studies, a progressive research-oriented NGO based in Rio de Janeiro, to produce *Fala Mulher da Vida* (*Speak, Woman, of the Life*), a manual designed to teach female sex workers to become peer educators. A study by ABIA explains the understandings underlying the project:

> It was expected that information on HIV prevention would pass from peer educators/agents to peer prostitutes and from prostitute to sexual partners and clients, and eventually to the larger population. The programme design was based on an epidemiological model, which aimed at impacting on 'vectors of transmission' as a strategy to multiply quality information on the epidemic but also contain infection rates. (Pimenta *et al.* 2010, p. 14)

The biopolitics underlying the notions of vectors of transmission, high-risk groups, and 'multiplying agents' are worth noting. Locating illness within territorialised populations that are clearly bounded yet whose boundaries are also porous, opening others to potential contagion, the project sought not just to limit contagion but to employ the 'vectors' themselves to transform the transmission of illness into the transmission of knowledge. NGOs were key because they could implement governmental action with populations and territories deemed hard-to-reach. If imperatives of effective governance provided an important basis for incipient networks, such networks did not represent a seamless web of biopolitical management or a single axis of power-knowledge, but rather, points of tension particularly about the kind of expert knowledge that should guide its course.

These tensions came to light in an article written by Gabriela Silva Leite (1989), then Coordinator of the Prostitution and Civil Rights programme. The piece was prompted when National programme officials rejected the materials produced by activists for failing to meet technical specifications on scientific content, citing, among other points, the lack of diagrammes showing HIV infecting human cells. Noting that 'official discourse can hide a range of prejudices, stigmas and discriminations, all in the name of "science"', Leite responded that her organisation's decision to participate in Previna was essentially a political one, explaining:

> We have worked for some years in the 'world of prostitution,' and we know that such groups have their own characteristics and cultures, which must be respected; we are also guided by evidence that when we train health professionals and multidisciplinary teams (trainers), we should prioritise knowledge of prostitution, as it is much more likely for these people to have knowledge about the nature of the virus than of all the social issues involved in prostitution.

Notably, Leite framed her political challenge to health officials' more clinical epidemiological approach to prevention as a competing claim to expertise. Examining AIDS activists' contestation of expert knowledge in the USA, Epstein (1996) has particularly stressed their acquired fluency in the language of biomedicine. Here, however, the claim to specialised knowledge is based primarily on activists' identification with target populations and consequent access to their 'characteristics and cultures', if anything inflected more by anthropology than biomedicine.[5] Ultimately, after a national meeting that brought together representatives of the Brazilian Prostitutes Network, *travesti* activists, and state officials, the National programme approved activists' material, essentially validating their approach. Like other programme activities, Previna came to a standstill with the economic crisis, to be retaken as Previna II after the infusion of World Bank funds.

The Bank's interest in capacity-building was directly related to its turn to NGOs as potential 'partners' in development in the 1980s and reflected a reconceptualisation of technologies of governmentality in relation to territory and expertise. In 1982, the Bank created an NGO-World Bank Committee, responding to widespread criticism of its policies by NGOs the previous decade (Petchesky 2003). In 1988, it issued an Operational Manual Statement establishing the first guidelines for collaboration with NGOs and published a discussion paper on the topic written by Cernea (1988). Cernea, the first sociologist to join the Bank's staff, had long advocated for the incorporation of anthropological and sociological expertise in development projects as a way of grounding them more firmly in local realities. 'The essence of the NGO approach', he explained, 'was not to induce development financially, but to mobilise people into organised structures of voluntary group action for self-reliance and self-development' (pp. 7–8). NGOs' 'comparative advantage' lay in their ability to: (1) promote local participation, thus mobilising and channelling social capacities; (2) operate at low cost, given their reliance on volunteerism; (3) innovate and adapt, as organisations unhampered by government bureaucracy; and (4) reach poor and remote areas in ways that, again, could incorporate knowledge of local realities while creating local 'stakeholders' to ensure the long-term sustainability of development efforts (pp. 17–18). The World Bank-NGO Committee led to the International Forum on Capacity-Building of Southern NGOs, an interagency body established in 1998.

The Bank's involvement in the Brazilian response marked a critical turning point for the National programme, channelling resources to permit its consolidation and significantly restructuring arrangements with NGOs. The First AIDS and STD Control Project, or AIDS I (1994–1998), aimed at improving epidemiological surveillance and prevention efforts, particularly among 'high-risk groups'. The US$250 million package (including $90 million in government funds) was conditioned on the incorporation of civil society as a key part of the national response. Justified largely on the basis of economic criteria, the Bank again pointed to NGOs' comparative advantage rooted both in a form of expertise – activists' 'specialised knowledge' of 'marginalised segments of society with which governments may have little experience' – and in their 'relationship of trust' with 'members of certain high-risk groups', in essence, their capacity to create an affective environment for effective (self-) governance.[6] It was also expected that NGO oversight would increase accountability, transparency, and effectiveness, performing a function of 'societal control', which resonated with the precepts of healthcare reformers and which National programme officials have increasingly prioritised in recent years. Such oversight, however, would operate in both directions (without extending to the Bank itself). Under the terms of the loan, a new competitive mechanism was created for NGO contracting, with external evaluation committees to assess proposals on the basis of managerial, epidemiological, and geographic criteria and NGOs themselves on criteria such as legal status, structure, technical capacity, and past experience. New oversight mechanisms also required quarterly progress reports and on-site visits by programme officials.[7]

The impact of these arrangements on civil society is by no means neutral. They have strengthened certain sectors of social movements over others, by channelling greater resources to larger, more established NGOs to the detriment of smaller ones; or in the case of LGBT activism, to gay men's and trans groups over lesbian organisations. They have also reinforced what the social anthropologist Galvão (2000), a former director of the NGO Articulation Unit, has termed the 'dictatorship of the projects', referring to forms of activism structured around the implementation of projects, constrained by limited time-horizons, and the production of quantifiable results. Indeed, the arrangements of mutual oversight built into these contracts are, in a sense, designed to operate as self-regulating panoptic networks, with each actor responsible for overseeing the other in the name of good governance. Potential tensions are thus incorporated into a rationality of government designed to discipline all the actors involved, though in ways inflected by relations of asymmetry, with NGOs in a position of economic dependence in a context of increasing competition. Subsequent loans expanded prevention efforts to new populations and areas beyond major cities; promoting the decentralisation of functions, including NGO contracting, to states and municipalities; and strengthening oversight mechanisms through increased demands for quantifiable outcomes. While the Bank's involvement marked a clear turning point in the course of AIDS policy, the Brazilian government played an important role mediating the terms of this arrangement. In part reflecting tensions embedded in policy networks, the Bank, indeed, disagreed with important aspects of Brazilian AIDS and healthcare policy, including its international advocacy of access to medications as a human right superseding intellectual property, its 1996 law guaranteeing universal access to AIDS drugs, and more generally its constitutional framing of healthcare as a social right (Mattos et al. 2001, Ramos 2004).

On the questions of civic participation and decentralisation, however, Bank prescriptions found resonance not just with the demands of healthcare activists but with the project of state restructuring of the Fernando Henrique Cardoso administration (1995–2002). Influenced by international currents advocating a 'third way' – an effort to reinvent social democracy by rearticulating the social safety net through neoliberal technologies of governmentality – the administration issued a General Plan to Reform the State Apparatus in 1995, announcing a new 'managerial' form of public administration based on principles of efficiency and productivity. Under the model, the federal government would devolve functions in 'non-strategic' areas like culture, health, and education to other levels of government, the private sector, and civil society organisations, now framed as the 'public non-state sector'. For its part, the federal government would shift its emphasis from the means of delivering social policies to measurable outcomes produced through contractual relations, primarily occupying a regulatory and coordinating role (Câmara da Reforma do Estado 1995). Cardoso would later recall: 'I always said that we needed to have a porous state so that society could act in it. The case of AIDS is the maximum (sic.): the state and the social movement practically fused' (Biehl 2004, p. 115).

In the area of AIDS prevention, capacity-building became a key technology for realising this vision, expressed in a series of projects designed to extend the territorial and demographic reach of activism and consequently of public policy. In 1999, the National programme launched the SOMOS Project in partnership with the Brazilian Gay, Lesbian, Bisexual, Travesti, and Transsexual Association (ABGLT). Four, and later six more established NGOs with the ABGLT were designated 'regional advocacy and training centres'. Through workshops and follow-up visits, these centres were responsible for strengthening smaller NGOs doing prevention work with MSMs and promoting the creation of new ones within their territories. Training encompassed four broad areas: (1) interventions, training activists to become peer educators with MSMs to encourage safe sex; (2) institutional development, involving such skills as how to legally register an organisation, create statutes, and write project proposals; (3) advocacy, involving skills like lobbying for antidiscrimination legislation and handling cases of homophobia; and (4) creating favourable environments, involving skills in public relations, media communications, and relations with other institutions.[8]

As a technology of governmentality, SOMOS is notable for the scope of relations it seeks to regulate. Informed by a transnational paradigm shift that expanded the purview of prevention from the individual behaviour within 'high-risk groups' to structural conditions increasing vulnerability to infection (Altman 2007), SOMOS framed combating homophobia, both societal and internalised, as the key to prevention. In doing so, it folded into governance both macro-structural factors, in its focus on advocacy and favourable environments, and the most intimate sphere of subject formation, by linking prevention to the exercise of citizenship and the promotion of self-esteem. As the ABGLT explains: 'The philosophy of the SOMOS Project is based on the principle that the full exercise of citizenship is the essential element for STD/AIDS Prevention'. To confront homophobia, the project:

> Believes that training and strengthening organised groups of MSM who act to promote citizenship can be a way of reversing the situation. Working to reduce prejudice and discrimination towards homosexuality, the groups facilitate a process of interaction with the society in general and contribute to strengthening the self-esteem of the people involved, thus reflected in the prevention process: HE WHO LOVES HIMSELF TAKES CARE OF HIMSELF.[9]

This emphasis on self-esteem, evident in capacity-building projects in AIDS prevention throughout the 1990s, extends their scope beyond the transmission of skills, information, and resources prioritised in early projects, to encompass practices of self designed to induce deeper transformations at the level of subjectivity and affect. According to political theorist Cruikshank (1996, pp. 232–234), by turning the 'relationship of self-to-self' into a relationship that is governable, self-esteem becomes a 'technology in the sense that it is a specialised knowledge of how to esteem our selves, to estimate, calculate, measure, evaluate, discipline, and judge ourselves'. While the individualising implications of this focus on self-esteem are evident, its linkage to citizenship implies an understanding that, far from private, turns it into a social obligation, calling on 'citizen-subjects' to govern themselves in particular ways, 'so that the police, the guards, and the doctors do not have to'. Reflecting the changing contours of citizenship in the context of neoliberal globalisation, networks of disparate actors thus seek to optimise subjectivities by eliciting individuals' capacities to claim rights, challenge homophobia, and adhere to medical prescriptions (Ong 2006).

The National programme subsequently replicated the SOMOS model with other populations, launching the Maria Sem Vergonha Project in 2002, in partnership with the Brazilian Prostitutes Network; the Tulipa Project in 2004, in partnership with the National Travesti and Transsexual Articulation (ANTRA); and the Roda Brasil Project in 2007, targeting intravenous drug users, in partnership with the Brazilian Harm Reducers Association (ABORDA). The continuities of the model from the Cardoso to the Lula administration, and to some extent with earlier projects dating to Previna, again speak to a dimension of capacity-building – and indeed, of a contemporary, medicalised sexual politics – operating less at the level of overt (i.e. partisan) ideology than as a modular technology of governmentality, deployable across ideological contexts.[10]

We have sought to trace the gradual institutionalisation of this technology in Brazil through policy networks, which came together in part because disparate projects advanced by different actors – activists, state officials, and the World Bank – overlapped in calls for civic participation and decentralisation. Against the transnational backdrop discussed above, this overlap laid the basis for the so-called Brazilian response, which has itself, as a former National programme director observed, become an 'exportable Brazilian product' (Castro and Bernadete da Silva 2005, p. 283). The implications of these developments for social movements are ambiguous. Very clearly, the biopolitical constitution 'vulnerable populations' has legitimised social actors and causes that once would have been dismissed as deviant. In some instances, this has allowed activists to expand regulatory frameworks, as in their fight for access to medicines or challenges to the narrow epidemiological paradigm initially guiding Previna, discussed above. At the same time, to the extent that the path to liberation and the path to regulation become one and the same, these frameworks have also constrained and channelled activism through particular institutional paths while also fostering relations of financial dependence. The growing delegation of AIDS contracting to states and municipalities as part of a larger project of decentralisation has particularly underscored the latter point, as many NGOs have found their sources of funding declining.

Conclusion

This article traces the multi-stranded genealogy of capacity-building as a technology of governmentality widely deployed in projects of HIV/AIDS prevention. In particular, we highlighted its institutionalisation through policy networks articulating multiple actors and its complex genealogy, presenting tensions and conflicts that nevertheless are potentially productive and inherent to such networks. The use of this technology to govern HIV/AIDS reflects, in part, the pandemic's emergence at a time of neoliberal ascendance. Beyond a liberalisation of markets and a retraction of labour protections and other pillars of the welfare state, as Foucault (2008) observed, neoliberalism also produced new technologies of government that rely on regulatory arrangements designed to mobilise the vitality and capacities of populations towards reflexive self-government. For some groups once marginalised, such technologies have opened unprecedented opportunities to claim citizenship and social rights, especially the right to healthcare, through a curious intermingling of a politics of recognition, subjectification and optimisation. Indeed, for particularly stigmatised groups (*travestis*; sex workers), HIV/AIDS programmes often represent the only official doorways opened. This recasting of guarantees of citizenship through policy networks reconfigures historic boundaries between civil society and the state, public and private, national and transnational, and democratic representation and bureaucratic administration (Ong 2006). In focusing on these dimensions, this paper also seeks to demonstrate the relevance of Foucauldian notions of governmentality and biopower to social scientific analyses of the HIV/AIDS pandemic.

Finally, we considered the multi-stranded genealogy of capacity-building at both the international level and in Brazil, thus seeking: to highlight the resilience of national actors in mediating international prescriptions (perhaps more forceful in Brazil given the size of its economy and its geopolitical weight); to offer an understanding of policy networks as arenas marked by asymmetries but where power does also circulate actively and in productive ways; and to suggest the modular and mutable nature of the neoliberal arts of government. In Brazil, more than many other countries, notions of popular participation and universal access have guided healthcare policies in general, particularly in the area of HIV/AIDS, and the 'Brazilian response' has, in a sense, grafted these precepts onto neoliberal formulas. The tremendously productive integration of civil society, state, and transnational players in Brazil's HIV/AIDS policy networks has thus produced a tense and complex balance of the most fundamental, intimate human needs with large and impersonal market forces and the changing claims-making positions of all those involved, from state administrators to activists to those beyond the boundaries of networks, on the margins of civic life. Governmentality and biopower offer a critical lens to understand these dynamics, as they really exist, and therefore to comment, hopefully in a useful manner, on these processes.

Notes

1. Foucault (1991) traces a shift in early modernity away from a politics of domination associated with sovereign power, towards a governmental power emphasising the administration of people's conduct towards the collective good.
2. While including social movement organisations and often claiming the mantle of representation, policy networks differ from traditional social movements because their potentially heterogeneous composition straddles historic boundaries between state and civil society; public and private, and differ from traditional interest groups because of their role not just pressing for but also implementing public policies. As we elaborate below, HIV/AIDS work has been marked by the breadth and intricacy of these networks working across sectors locally, nationally, and globally.
3. http://www.un.org/esa/dsd/agenda21/res_agenda21_37.shtml.
4. In Portuguese, 'capacity building' can be translated as 'construção de capacidades', though in this paper, we also consider projects using related terminology, including *multiplicadores*, or peer-educators, and *fortalecimento/desenvolvimento institucional*, or institutional strengthening/development.
5. Medical anthropologists came to play an increasingly important role in both activist and official circles at about this time. Similarly challenging the universalising categories of epidemiology, they stressed the importance of attention to the meanings and erotic practices circulating in discrete (if at times exoticised) 'sexual cultures' (Víctora and Knauth 2002).
6. 'Brazil: Third AIDS and STD Control Project: Project Information Document PID11512', World Bank, 15 November 2002.

7. 'Sector and thematic evaluation group and operations evaluation department. Report no. 28819. Project performance assessment report: Brazil First and Second AIDS and STD Control Projects (Loan 3659-BR and 4392-BR)', World Bank, 27 April 2004.
8. *Juntos somos mais fortes*. Curitiba: ABGLT, 2003.
9. *Juntos somos mais fortes*, pp. 18–19.
10. While the National programme's support contributed significantly to the scope of these projects, it is also worth underscoring that quite similar initiatives have been carried out in Brazil and elsewhere without significant state involvement and with nongovernmental sources of funds, again speaking to the flexible nature of the policy networks involved in capacity-building and AIDS prevention.

References

Altman, D., 1994. *Power and community: organizational and cultural responses to AIDS*. London: Taylor & Francis.
Altman, D., 2007. Rights matter: structural interventions and vulnerable communities. *Interamerican Journal of Psychology*, 41 (1), 87–92.
Biehl, J., 2004. The activist state: global pharmaceuticals, AIDS, and citizenship in Brazil. *Social Text*, 22 (3), 105–132.
Burchell, G., 1996. Liberal government and techniques of the self. *In*: A. Barry, T. Osborne and N. Rose, eds. *Foucault and political reason: liberalism, neo-liberalism, and rationalities of government*. Chicago: University of Chicago Press, 19–36.
Câmara da Reforma do Estado, 1995. *Plano diretor da reforma do aparelho do estado*. Brasilia: Presidência da República.
Câmara da Silva, C.L., 1998. ONGs/AIDS, intervenções sociais e novos laços de solidariedade social. *Cadernos de Saúde Pública*, 14 (2), 129–139.
Campbell, C., 2003. *'Letting them Die': why HIV/AIDS prevention programmes fail*. Bloomington: Indiana University Press.
Campos, L.C.M., 2005. *Estado e terceiro setor na prestação de serviços públicos: O programmea Nacional de DST/AIDS*. Masters Thesis in Government and Public Administration. São Paulo: Fundação Getúlio Vargas-Escola de Administração de Empresas de São Paulo.
Castro, M.G. and Bernadete da Silva, L., 2005. *Responses to AIDS challenges in Brazil: limits and possibilities*. Brasilia: UNESCO, Ministry of Health.
Cernea, M., 1988. *Nongovernmental organizations and local development*. World Bank Discussion Papers, no. 40. Washington, DC: The World Bank.
Chalmers, D.A., Martin, S.B., and Piester, K., 1997. Associative networks: new structures of representation for the popular sectors? *In*: D.A. Chalmers, C.M. Vilas, K. Hite, S.B. Martin, K. Piester and M. Segarra, eds. *The new politics of inequality in Latin America: rethinking participation and representation*. Oxford: Oxford University Press, 543–592.
Chambre, S., 2006. *Fighting for our lives: New York's AIDS community and the politics of disease*. New Brunswick: Rutgers University Press.
CICT, 2008. *La Cooperación sur-sur en el contexto de la epidemia del SIDA: Tres años del Centro de Cooperación Técnica Internacional en VIH/SIDA*. Brasilia: Ministério de Saúde.
Cruikshank, B., 1996. Revolutions within: self-government and self-esteem. *In*: A. Barry, T. Osborne and N. Rose, eds. *Foucault and political reason: liberalism, neo-liberalism, and rationalities of government*. Chicago: University of Chicago Press, 231–251.
Daniel, H., 1994. *Vida antes da morte*. Rio de Janeiro: ABIA.
Davida, 1998. Prostituição, direitos civis, saúde. Encontro de Lideranças da Rede Nacional de Profissionais do Sexo: Relatório.
de la Dehesa, R., 2010. *Queering the public sphere in Mexico and Brazil: sexual rights movements in emerging democracies*. Durham, NC: Duke University Press.
Eade, D., 1997. *Capacity-building: an approach to people-centred development*. Oxford: Oxfam Publishing.
Epstein, S., 1996. *Impure science: AIDS, activism, and the politics of knowledge*. Berkeley, CA: University of California Press.
Farmer, P., 2004. *Pathologies of power: health, human rights, and the new war on the poor*. Berkeley, CA: University of California Press.

Fleury, S., 1997. A questão democrática na saúde. In: S. Fleury, ed. *Saúde e democracia: A luta dos CEBES*. São Paulo: Lemos Editorial, 25–41.

Foucault, M., 1991. Governmentality. In: G. Burchell, C. Gordon and P. Miller, eds. *The Foucault effect: studies in governmentality: with two lectures by and an interview with Michel Foucault*. Chicago: University of Chicago Press, 87–104.

Foucault, M., 2008. *The birth of biopolitics: lectures at the Collège de France, 1978–79* (G. Burchell, trans.). New York: Palgrave-Macmillan.

Gabriela Silva Leite, 1989. *Impasse no Projeto Previna: Entre a vida e a célula. Boletim*, no. 8. Rio de Janeiro: ABIA.

Galvão, J., 2000. *AIDS no Brasil: a agenda de construção de uma epidemia*. Rio de Janeiro: ABIA.

George, S., 2004. *Another world is possible if...* New York: Verso Books.

Granjeiro, A., Laurinda da Silva, L., and Teixeira, P.R., 2009. Resposta à AIDS no Brasil. *Revista Panamericana de Salud Pública*, 26 (1), 87–94.

Grebe, E., 2008. *Transnational networks of influence in South African AIDS treatment activism*. Centre for Social Science Research Working Paper No. 222. Capetown, South Africa. Available from: http://www.cssr.uct.ac.za/sites/cssr.uct.ac.za/files/pubs/WP222.pdf [accessed 20 June 2011].

Guta, A., Flicker, S., and Roche, B., 2011. Critically reflecting on the use of 'peer researchers' in community-based participatory research. Foucault Society: 2011 Colloquium Series. CUNY, New York, 4 May.

Jana, S., et al., 2004. The Sonagachi project: a sustainable community intervention programme. *AIDS Education and Preventio*, 16 (5), 405–414.

Keck, M. and Sikkink, K., 1998. *Activists beyond borders: advocacy networks in international politics*. Ithaca, NY: Cornell University Press.

Mattos, R.A., Terto, V., Jr., and Parker, R., 2001. *As estratégias do Banco Mundial e a resposta à AIDS no Brasil*. Rio de Janeiro: ABIA.

Ministerio da Saúde, 2002. *Profissionais do sexo: Documento referencial para ações de prevenção das DST e da AIDS*. Brasilia: Secretaria de Políticas de Saúde, Coordenação Nacional de DST e AIDS.

Ong, A., 2006. *Neoliberalism as exception: mutations in citizenship and sovereignty*. Durham, NC: Duke University Press.

Patton, C., 1990. *Inventing AIDS*. New York: Routledge.

Petchesky, R.P., 2003. *Global prescriptions: gendering health and human rights*. London: Zed Books, in association with the United Nations Research Institute for Social Development.

Pimenta, C., et al., 2010. *Sexuality and development: Brazil's national response to HIV/AIDS amongst sex workers*. Rio de Janeiro: ABIA.

Ramos, S., 2004. O papel das ONGs na construção de políticas de saúde: A Aids, a saúde da mulher, e a saúde mental. *Ciência y Saúde Coletiva*, 9 (4), 1067–1078.

Torres-Ruiz, A., 2011. HIV/AIDS and sexual minorities in Mexico: a globalised struggle for the protection of human rights. *Latin American Research Review*, 46 (1), 30–53.

Treichler, P., 1999. *How to have theory in an epidemic: cultural chronicles of AIDS*. Durham, NC: Duke University Press.

Víctora, C.G. and Knauth, D.R., 2002. Entrevista com Richard Parker. *Horizontes Antropológicos*, 8 (17), 253–262.

Constitution, diversification and normalization of a health problem: organizing the fight against AIDS in Switzerland (1984–2005)

Michael Voegtli and Olivier Fillieule

The article traces the formation, diversification and normalization of the AIDS cause in Switzerland. Particular emphasis is placed on interactions between the medical field, public authorities and associative space, the latter being understood as the place where individual and collective actors compete to define the cause. The authors argue that the major phases in the structuring of the struggle, the pace of state intervention and the creation of a multi-organizational field, can only be understood if one adopts a 'configurational perspective' attentive to the manner in which, in a given context and under the effect of particular constraints, key actors strategically interact and contribute to transforming their environment and their chances of reaching their goals. This approach takes into account the changing socio-biological characteristics of those who have committed themselves to the cause. In turn, internal movement divisions about how to respond to the epidemic as well as the changing perceptions of the disease have modified the opportunities for commitment, encouraging certain individual kinds of people and excluding others.

Introduction

It is often challenging to ascertain the construction and transformation of causes. In the fight against AIDS in Switzerland the construction of responses to the epidemic and their successive transformations since 1984, particularly during the period known as 'normalization', may only be understood through correlating the organization of the struggle with the social characteristics of activists (both volunteers and professionals). These successive waves of activist involvement have served to shape the responses to the epidemic. Battles amongst activists during the transformation of the epidemic's public image affected the possibilities for involvement, thus permitting us to explain the participation, persistence and withdrawal of various activists.

We reject the perspective of a heterogeneity of causes (much earlier determinants, and initial states) and their effects (the various forms of mobilization and their results). Instead, we suggest an examination of causal chains, the processes by which individual acts and the structures of action are set in place and are modified as a result of strategic interactions. Thus we adopt a processual perspective, attentive to the manner in which, in a given context and under the effect of particular constraints, the actors, strategically interact, and contribute to transforming their environment and their objective chances of reaching their goals. In such a model, activism is conceived as a long-lasting social activity articulated by phases of joining, commitment, and defection (Whittier 1997, Fillieule 2001, 2010). Our theoretical approach is in line with the concept of 'configuration', denoting a dynamic pattern in articulating different scales of analysis, that was coined by Elias (1939, 1970) when describing certain patterns of relations between human beings (figuration in German).[1]

This paper considers the interactions between the medical field, public authorities and associative space in the fight against AIDS, the latter being understood as the place where individual and collective actors compete to define the cause. Indeed, integrating these three spaces allows us to show how the public image of HIV/AIDS has been transformed (Pinell *et al.* 2002) and how this impacts on the possibilities for participation. This demonstrates the evolution of the AIDS problem from the beginnings of 'exceptionalism' (Kirp and Bayer 1992) to the phase of 'normalization' (Kübler *et al.* 2002, Rosenbrock *et al.* 2000) on the basis of the transformation of the public problem, In fact, as Setbon (2000, p. 63) emphasizes:

> It is not the problem which changes as an effect of the responses, but its perception and social acceptability that are modified by the exceptional responses, by the advances, however limited, in AIDS therapies, and, more broadly, by the uncertainty which characterized the mobilization phase. Together this creates a new depiction of the problem, provides the public with preventive measures and makes the risk more acceptable.

These notions of 'normalization' and 'exceptionalism' are 'scientific categories', as well as 'practical categories', used both by scientists, to describe all the developments in the fight against the epidemic, and actors who invest time and energy in the anti-AIDS fight. The definition of normalization is itself one of the issues at stake in the struggle. As a scientific category, normalization refers to the process of institutionalization of the social movement of the fight against AIDS, the transformation of the AIDS problem from a major danger to a controllable problem and the corresponding retreat of public authorities, with AIDS losing its central character on the public health agenda.

The article is based on research focusing on participation in the fight against AIDS in Switzerland (at the federal level and in seven federated states – cantons).[2] We begin by showing the basis of the initial response to the epidemic and the form it assumed. Then, we focus on the aspects contributing to modifying the cause at the end of the 1980s. Finally, we discuss the impact of the introduction of HAART on the redefinition of the fight against AIDS in Switzerland.

The formation of an initial response

As in most countries (Altman 1994), when AIDS arrived in Switzerland, the initial framing associated the illness with male homosexuality. The debate that subsequently occurred in homosexual organizations was to determine whether they prioritize the issue, thereby running the risk of redoubling the stigma attached to the gay community. This issue was rapidly resolved in favour of active participation. While the 1970s had seen tensions between homophile groups (the main one being the Organization suisse des homophiles – SOH (the Swiss Organization of Homophiles)) and homosexual working groups, brought together within the Coordination homosexuelle suisse (CHOSE – Swiss Homosexual Coordination), the start of the 1980s was marked by greater collaboration. The costs and the risks (Wiltfang and McAdam 1991) of involvement in homosexual liberation groups, particularly the high visibility that they demanded of their members, prevented wider recruitment. Gradually, in a similar fashion to what Armstrong (2002), in particular, revealed in the case of the USA, mobilization became less radical and more sectorial, giving rise to new groups or a transformation of activist philosophy within existing associations towards more of an identity model (Gay Identity).

These associations also remain the only ones to publish a specialized gay press and be connected to the most visible social gathering spots. The gay commercial scene was, by comparison, small. There is not unlike in France, for example (Pinell et al. 2002), a specialized press or a commercial centre large enough to compete with Swiss associations, that remain dominant in determining the orientation of the fight that the 'homosexual community' must lead. In other words, while it is true, as Duyvendak (1995) claims, that at the time when the AIDS epidemic emerged, there was a solid foundation of homosexual movements at the local level, it is incorrect to claim that these movements were fragmented, with little national presence. The movements are mostly represented in one of two umbrella organizations, CHOSE or SOH, and often collaborate. This point is important, because when the epidemic appeared, the people involved in the associations were capable of providing a rapid response to this new threat.

The creation of the Swiss Aids Federation

Homosexual activists received substantial support from the recently named director of the epidemiological section of the FOPH, Bertino Somaini. Somaini proved to be one of the principal architects of rapprochement of public authorities and homosexual groups. Before being named to the FOPH, he was engaged in post-graduate study at the University of California, Berkeley. It was at Berkeley that Somaini first heard of AIDS. He also witnessed the initial organizing of the American homosexual movement. He combined what he learned from this experience with the Swiss administrative approach to social problems:

> The homosexuals in San Francisco were very well organized, and therefore it was a hundred times better to let a private organization act rather than have the authorities intervene. [...]. So we, the state, we said: 'we will finance you, but only if you get together' [...]. There was no direct pressure from the state; there was the experience of what happens when the state wants an organization like the FOPH to intervene. [...] The state supports an umbrella organization and, after that, it works, parliament comes up with the money. This is the administrative approach. So, I followed it. (Somaini interview)

To avoid dispersal of resources, Somaini suggested that AIDS delegates create a unified organization as quickly as possible, stressing that the FOPH could only associate with preventative actions in the field of AIDS if the structure that it might support was sufficiently generalist. This would allow for the widespread dissemination of HIV prevention messages to the entire population and unite people active in other groups who were also strongly affected by HIV/AIDS notably sex workers and social workers dealing with drug users.

AIDS delegates of homosexual working groups first attempted to coordinate their actions and then present a united front before the FOPH. From this dual perspective, they chose to establish the first organization, named AIDS-Hilfe Schweiz (Swiss Help Against AIDS). Three people played a pivotal role in its conception: Marcel Ulmann, president of SOH, Herbert Riedener, president of the Zurich 'leather association', Loge 70, and Roger Staub, member of the Zurich gay liberation group (HAZ). Given the urgency of the situation, and putting aside the dissensions amongst the gay associations concerning AIDS, all three volunteers defended an approach favouring rapid intervention in the field of prevention.

On 2 June 1985, the Swiss Aids Federation (Aide Suisse contre le sida/AIDS-Hilfe Schweiz – SAF) was officially founded in Zurich at an assembly bringing together fourteen homosexual associations. The FOPH also became a member, which was unprecedented: this was the first time that a state organization belonged to a private association, not to mention a organization founded by homosexuals. The first president of SAF was the television journalist André Ratti. At the opening of SAF's first press conference on 2 July 1985, he declared: 'My name is

André Ratti. I am homosexual myself, I am 50 years old, and since April I have known that I have AIDS'. The conference served to remind the public that gays were not the only ones affected, and neither were drug users or sex workers. The entire population was ultimately at risk of contracting the disease. Nonetheless, there was no minimization of the heavy toll on homosexuals, and the fight has remained closely linked to homosexuality.

It is important to highlight that the situation in Switzerland was different to most other places in Europe, and particularly France and the UK, concerning the way in which the anti-AIDS campaign was organized. Switzerland is closer to that of the USA or Australia (Kippax et al. 1993, Altman 1994). In France, the association AIDES was a unifying force, with the sick individual firmly at the centre of their concerns: 'from this [comes] a movement that, in putting sick people at the heart of their concerns, does not organizationally link the fight against AIDS to the gay community, but rather establishes itself as a space to unite those who are sick and all those who are concerned about the epidemic' (Pinell et al. 2002, pp. 47–48). In Germany, the perspective adopted during the founding of Deutsche Aids-Hilfe was also one of offering support to those who were ill (Schilling 2000). Putting the illness at the centre of the mobilization effort, in France for example, meant that, very rapidly, there was both dehomosexualization (the distinction between AIDS and homosexuality) and heterosexualization (an influx of heterosexual activists into the associations). As Staub underscored concerning the different approaches:

> One has to observe that Deutsche Aids Hilfe was created in 83 already, but to help and provide support to the sick. For us, this was not the case at all. [...] So, SAF has taken a different path [...]. We were a prevention agency based on the groups affected. This made for a strong concept. (Staub interview)

Activists agreed on the question of *prevention*, and this was the basis for the initial actions of SAF's local offices, showing that the way a cause is built contributes to how subsequent initiatives unfold. The division of responsibilities within the Swiss federal state means that it is largely up to the cantons to lead the fight against health problems within their territory. The creation of cantonal associations (local offices) was only to obtain financing to fight against AIDS and to work closely with the affected groups. In all the cantons where homosexual groups were active, they supported the creation of SAF local offices. SAF placed their infrastructure at the disposal of cantons with active homosexual groups, and members participated on a volunteer basis to ensure the prevention work continued. Thus, where homosexual groups existed, organizational and individual networks allowed for the rapid creation of local associations to fight against AIDS.

It is not possible to describe all the actions organized by SAF and various local groups in the field of prevention, as well as their support for affected individuals. It is sufficient to mention some of the most prominent, including promotion of condom use amongst the gay community, battles for anonymous HIV testing, for the maintenance of health insurance coverage for those whom insurers excluded due to their HIV-positive status, for access to new treatments and rapid listing as 'special treatments' (allowing for a reimbursement from the health insurance board), and for decent hospital conditions for the sick.

All these actions were, at the outset, undertaken on a volunteer basis, mostly by homosexual men who were involved because of their closeness to the illness, either because they were themselves affected (direct proximity), because they knew people who were ill (affective proximity) or because they identified with people with AIDS (cognitive proximity). Gradually, these activists were joined by others with a distinct vision of the nature of the fight against AIDS. This situation gave rise to numerous tensions culminating in the departure of the first wave of activists.

Changes at the heart of associations in the fight against AIDS and the tendency for homosexuals to withdraw

Three elements contributed to transforming the face of the fight in Switzerland and to the withdrawal of a first wave of homosexual activists from the associations. First, the initial results of the ELISA test in 1985 showed that homosexual men were not the only ones affected by the epidemic. The involvement of public authorities, at the federal level and in the cantons, also became more apparent. In particular, financing the fight against the spread of HIV increased very significantly starting from 1987 (900,000 Swiss francs, i.e. double the amount of the previous year). Finally, the campaign STOP AIDS was launched in February 1987, and it also encouraged the transformation of the epidemic's public image, by showing that it hit the entire population.

Archives and interviews, as well as responses to our quantitative survey, clearly showed that those first involved in the fight, mostly homosexual men, were joined first by heterosexual women, and then heterosexual men often because of their involvement in social services. This coexistence was not without its problems, because newcomers and long-time activists disagreed, particularly regarding the objectives and priorities of the fight against AIDS. Thus, crises erupted in the new umbrella organization and in many local offices as the following article, published at the end of 1987, demonstrates:

> The determining factor in current dissension is that AIDS has become a political matter. Suddenly, federal money for prevention is in the millions, and, with the FOPH, a major federal office was looking for an alliance with SAF. In the wake of this development, it became increasingly difficult for the Swiss Aids Federation to reconcile homosexuals', doctors,' politicians' and administrative officials' divergent interests and demands. To these, groups previously little or badly represented (drug specialists, and women) were added to the structures of the organization. The first line of combatants, coming from the homosexual scene, suddenly saw themselves involved in internal fights for power and prestige. (Tages Anzeiger, 14 November 1987)

These developments led to an initial professionalization within the associations due to the arrival of health and social workers. They also again resulted in a questioning of the authority of those first gay participants. Many homosexual activists left the SAF and its local offices, some returning to homosexual working groups. This tendency could be clearly seen in interviews with activists and ex-activists, as well as in the archives of gay associations. Our quantitative investigation offers a graphic illustration of this trend (Figure 1).

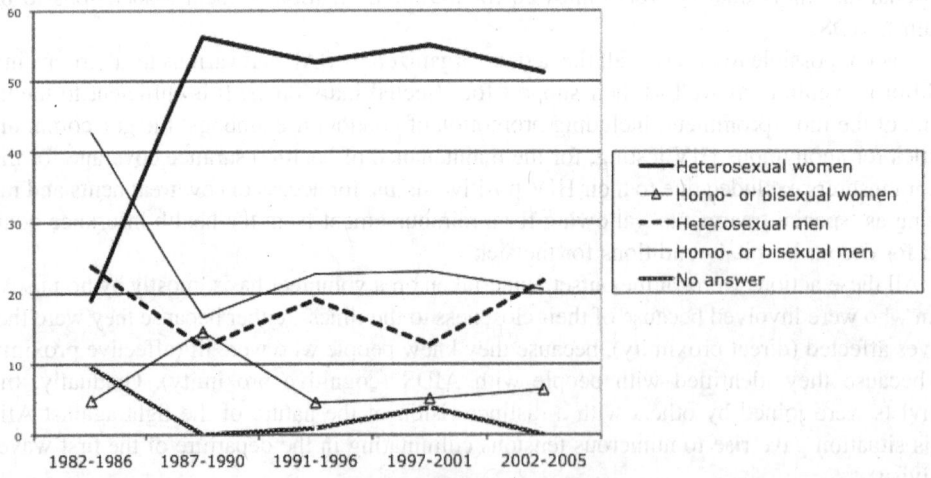

Figure 1. Respondents' sex and socio-sexual orientation (in percentage terms for each phase).

These quantitative data also confirms our conclusions gained from other sources about the fight against AIDS, namely, that homosexual men, a majority up until 1986, were joined in the movement by heterosexual women. Often as part of their training in the social or health sectors, these women participated in developing recreational activities suitable for different stages of the illness. Thus, prevention was no longer the central focus. At the organizational level, the separation between homosexual associations and local offices of SAF became increasingly apparent. There was also a distinct separation of activities between anti-AIDS organizations and homosexual associations, with subtle variations, in practically all the cantons.

It is clear that male homosexuals increasingly did volunteer work in the fight against the epidemic, but the process of dehomosexualization of AIDS and heterosexualization of populations active within the associations continued in subsequent years, culminating in the middle of 1996.

Changes in the fight against the epidemic: the 'normalization' of HIV/AIDS

From the summer of 1996, and with the widespread availability in Switzerland of HAART, the fight against AIDS changed considerably. Above all, there was a significant drop in mortality and morbidity. There was also a further tendency towards the professionalization that began at the end of the 1980s, placing the fight against AIDS fully in the 'normalization' phase. In other words, as Rosenbrock *et al.* (2000, p. 1608) noted, the period was characterized by a change in status of AIDS: 'In Europe – and with differences in all the wealthy countries – an impending catastrophe has turned into a problem that can be managed by public health and medical care'.

The trend described by Rosenbrock *et al.* dramatically changed the anti-AIDS cause and ways of being involved in it. The links between public authorities and actors in the associative spaces were considerably transformed. This period was characterized by a decline in public authorities' attention to AIDS. The most symptomatic dimension of the normalization process was the FOPH's intention to dissolve SAF, transferring responsibilities and structures and eventually reintegrating the HIV/AIDS into more mainstream public health organizations. The evolution of the number of people affected by the epidemic certainly had an effect on the diminution of public financing allocated to the fight against AIDS. Indeed, in Figure 2, we observe that the Confederation expenditures oscillated for the first part of the 1990s between approximately 13 million francs in 1990 and 15 million francs in 1996, peaking at almost 16 million in 1994. Over the course of the following years, the credits allocated to the fight consistently decreased, down to slightly more than 9.5 million francs in 2001, a third less than five years earlier.

Nonetheless, the epidemiological data must also be situated in the political context of the reduction in expenditures starting from the 1980s, which affected the policies of the Confederation from the mid 1990s on. This orientation is evident in the new Law on the organization of government and administration, of 1997. The law 'introduces the notion of term benefits that the Federal Council could transfer to certain administrative units, which will function according to the principles of new public management' (FF 1996, p. 17). Conceived on the basis of New Public Management (NPM) principles (Giauque 2003) it must allow, according to its promoters, the Confederation to limit its operational costs, to propose more efficient management and to decrease federal expenses.

Policies to fight AIDS were not spared from administrative reorganization and decreased public financing. Nevertheless, the introduction of NPM alone does not entirely explain the decline in resources. Indeed, while AIDS financing dropped between 1996 and 2001, money relating to general HIV prevention remained stable, even increasing at the end of the period. We could suppose that the decrease was due to new perceptions of the epidemic, and to the rise of other major public health problems that emerged during this period ('the mad cow

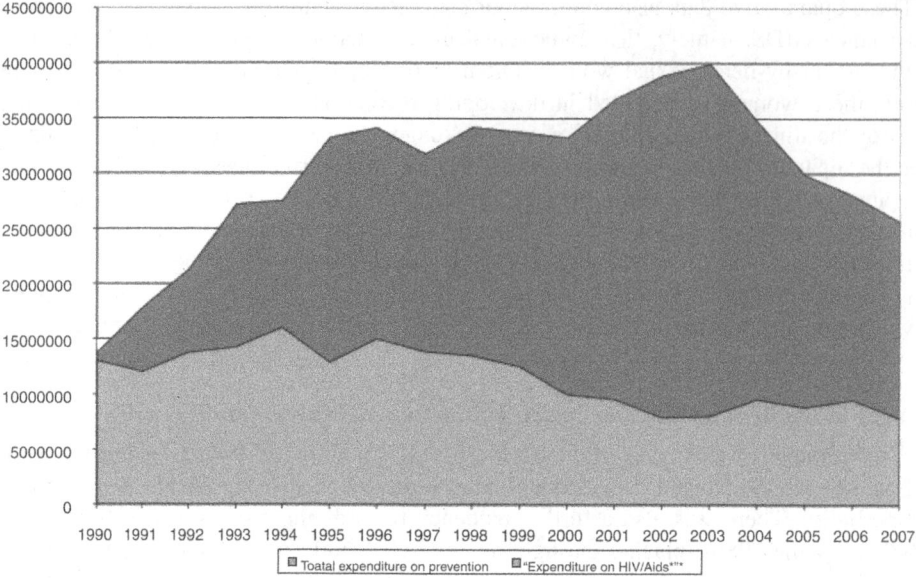

Figure 2. Evolution of the Confederation financing of the fight against AIDS.

crisis', and the fight against alcoholism and smoking). The evolution of public authorities' attention to the epidemic is, thus, directly linked to the transformation of the 'AIDS problem'.

Here, we reach an important point allowing us to focus on the mechanisms that change causes. It is not so much the characteristics of the phenomenon as how it is depicted that changes, and contributes to the perception of, the public problem. In the Swiss case, it is certainly this transformation of the problem that made public authorities consider that AIDS had become an 'acceptable risk', and which saw a decrease in public financing (from 16 millions francs in 1994 to 9.5 in 2001), in a context of limiting the cost of public finances. The new perception of the epidemic led to a series of transformations within the space of the fight against AIDS.

The effects of the transformation of the epidemic on the associative space of the fight against AIDS

The effects of this transformation are evident on a number of levels. First, the type of collaboration between the FOPH and SAF, allowing activists a considerable freedom in their actions, was questioned. This situation gradually evolved over the 1990s, and the widespread use of subsidies linked to term benefits produced an increased role for the FOPH in the implementation of strategies in the fight against the epidemic.

Then, to partially counter the tendency to make SAF a formally part of federal administrative policy, SAF sought to increase its own financing. After a period up to 1992 when the proportion of its own funds declined, to settle at less than 10% of its total income, it then tended to rise. Indeed, this indicated a new direction in the association's financial strategy, to allow greater freedom in its actions. Between 1996 and 2001, the proportion of the SAF funds which were its own went from slightly more than 27% to 38.7%.

This tendency towards normalization, closely associated with the emergence of HAART, led to further professionalization of members at the coordinating level of SAF. This increased for three reasons. On one hand, HAART prompted certain activists to rethink their commitment to the fight, and some withdrew after being involved for many years. On the other hand, the

SAF leadership modified the selection criteria for members. In other words, affective or effective proximity to the epidemic was no longer conceived as sufficient for involvement. The association adopted recruitment principles based on the possession of officially recognized skills, usually through training in health and social services, as a member of the SAF committee at the time stressed:

> In 1997 we decided to change. We told ourselves that it is not necessarily those who feel called upon to do something and who are close to AIDS who are the best ones to work in this field. We said that certain qualifications and skills are also required if one wants to work in this sector. Being affected was a meaningful qualification too, because those concerned have experience with the illness and often knowledge that professionals lacked. But today, nobody thinks that this is sufficient anymore. So, other qualifications are needed. In addition, knowledge of the associations and the management process are required. Also, specialists' knowledge of HIV. (Interview with the SAF committee)

The third element resulting from the process of normalization and leading to professionalization was the development of fundraising activities, influencing in turn the search for professionals who could do this. Those equipped to fundraise or manage programmes and teams were favoured, as a member of the SAF leadership of the time said:

> I no longer know how many people were there at the start, but approximately twenty people worked together at the secretariat, along with external experts. Such an organization could only be run in a professional manner. And it was with professionals that one could organize fundraising. And this is fairly independent of the theme. This could be AIDS or HIV, cancer, or I don't know what. This has to be done by professionals. (Interview with the SAF leadership)

Here we see that the link to the people affected was considerably weakened between the 'exceptionalism' phase and the present phase of 'normalization'. This very gradual evolution at the end of the 1980s was due to the growth in budgets allocated to the association, the concentration of volunteer work on the ground in cantonal offices and the type of collaboration established with public authorities.

These transformations served to further reinforce the institutionalization of the social movement against AIDS at the highest level, in that SAF is now seen more as an organization implementing public health programmes largely determined within the FOPH. This trend can also be observed in the cantons.

Changing patterns at the cantonal level

The normalization phase within the cantonal structure was also characterized by a number of reorientations within associations, although the upheavals affected them differently. Here, we consider three dimensions. First, we see how therapeutic advances transformed social connections within associations. Secondly, we examine the evolution of local associations' financing to measure the decline in public financing. Thirdly, we attempt to grasp the impact of the transformation of the AIDS problem on the eventual withdrawal of volunteers. Less a massive wave of volunteer disengagement, the period beginning in 1997 until today has been characterized more by a restructuring of the rationale for participation in the struggle.

Impact of treatments on the people affected and restructuring social links within associations

As Broqua (2005, p. 296) stressed in his analysis of Act Up Paris, the impact of therapeutic advances includes 'two levels of apprehending the problem: the individual level of managing the illness (one's own or that of those close to you) and the collective level'. On an individual basis, for most of those affected, therapeutic advances resulted in significant physical improvements. Generally, for those who are HIV-positive, the new treatments combined to bring about a reexamination of their lives, causing them to reinvest in areas that they had up until this point neglected (notably the professional domain), either because of their state of health, or because their imminent death meant that, they had to be involved in what was considered most urgent, notably the fight against the epidemic.

Enhanced life expectancy and improvement in the state of health led to greater visibility of new concerns. Joining or rejoining the professional world raised the question of possible discrimination in hiring once again. More broadly, the decision of whether to reveal or conceal HIV-positive status resurfaced. This became still more complicated given the potentially greater number of those to whom one may reveal their status (both because the person has a greater life expectancy and because an improved state of health allows for involvement in an increased number of social subsets: professional, familial, affective, social, etc.). This become more complicated because, as Mellini *et al.* (2004, p. 156) stressed,

> the theory of the progression of the illness turns out to be no longer relevant in explaining the disclosure of one's HIV/AIDS. The asymptomatic phase now being of more or less of indefinite duration, the thesis according to which revealing the illness would take place when it became visible or when the person needed material or emotional support is null and void.

At the collective level, this development also posed a series of problems. In one association of HIV-positive individuals, a member observed that therapeutic advances had the effect of breaking the group's internal solidarity:

> I also felt that, while before, everyone was in the same situation, since 1996, there have been those for whom HAART worked, whom we offered instead lifelong assistance, they had plans, they had recreational activities, and, depending on their state of health, even a job. While, at the same time, others were experiencing very serious side-effects from the therapies, even dying because the therapy had no effect on them. And this led to a considerable diversification of the association's activities. Also, for the first time, within the association, among HIV-positive individuals who had always had a great sense of solidarity, for example, we felt tensions, uneasiness/suffering [...]. While undergoing the same treatment, some were doing well and some were not doing well at all; some were doing badly. We started to feel that things were less united. (Interview Sid'action)

This extract shows that the links within the movement were transformed due to the impact of treatments. Thus, solidarity within the group was dissolving because expectations of the association were no longer the same for everyone. While it is difficult to obtain accurate data on this phenomenon from individuals who are part of such groups, we may hypothesize that this 'inequality' regarding the illness could have led, in some cases, to a withdrawal of certain activists. In any case, it influenced the perception of solidarity within the associative movement and on the community dimension of the group. While earlier the consolidation of an '*entre-soi*' had a bearing, primarily on identification with a 'community of destiny' (Pollak 1988) where the support for another was encouraged by the imminence of death, therapeutic advances individualized the experience of the illness and limited the development of an 'esprit de corps' (Blumer 1951. On this dimension of the fight against AIDS, cf. Herzlich 2002). To this was added the difficulty of identifying someone or something responsible for the new situation: while it was possible to blame the 'wait-and-see' attitude of public authorities, given the diversity of individual reactions to treatments, any generalization proved impossible. More widely, all the actions of associations in the associative space of the fight against AIDS changed and, consequently, so too did the definition of the cause.

Decrease in cantonal public financing?

The process of 'normalization' led to a drop in federal financing. It is worth determining whether such a tendency can be observed in the cantons. For most of the local offices, financing has not diminished significantly since 1996. However, according to the cantons, it is the type of complementary financing of local offices that has changed, and they are still more reliant on fundraising activities. Conversely, we see that after a period of growth in financing up until 1992, financing stagnated in subsequent years. This is shown in the case of local SAF offices in the cantons of Berne (AHBe) and Bâle (AHbB) (Figure 3).

Up until 1992, public financing increased each year. For example, in the case of AHBe, cantonal financing between 1990 and 1991 more than doubled. In other words, the stabilization of public finances preceded the introduction of HAART, indicating that 'normalization' took place earlier.

Therefore, rather than a drop in cantonal financing, it seems that two trends affected the evolution of the local offices' work. These are the drop in donations, on one hand, that diminished the freedom of members in managing independent projects. On the other hand was the transfer of responsibilities of the Confederation to the cantons and the development of term benefits, which also limited the possibility of launching specific projects. This latter created greater uncertainty about the long-term status of financing – which might be reduced – meaning that a project would have to be abandoned. The transfer of Confederation responsibilities to the cantons led to a decrease in public financing available for the fight against the epidemic, contributing to financial instability at the level of cantonal offices, which became more dependent on private financing. Overall, the maintenance of cantonal subsidies could not completely compensate for the drop in federal credits. Consequently, it became more difficult for local offices to plan for the long term usage of funds and to innovate in responding to changes in the epidemic.

A withdrawal of volunteers in local associations?

The effect of normalization on the withdrawal of volunteers at the canton level is important. It is difficult to systematically evaluate the evolution of the number of volunteers in local offices, since the data are often incomplete. However, on the basis of the figures available we note a slight decrease in volunteer participation, observable in most SAF local offices. It also seems that participation has declined and activist turnover is considerable.

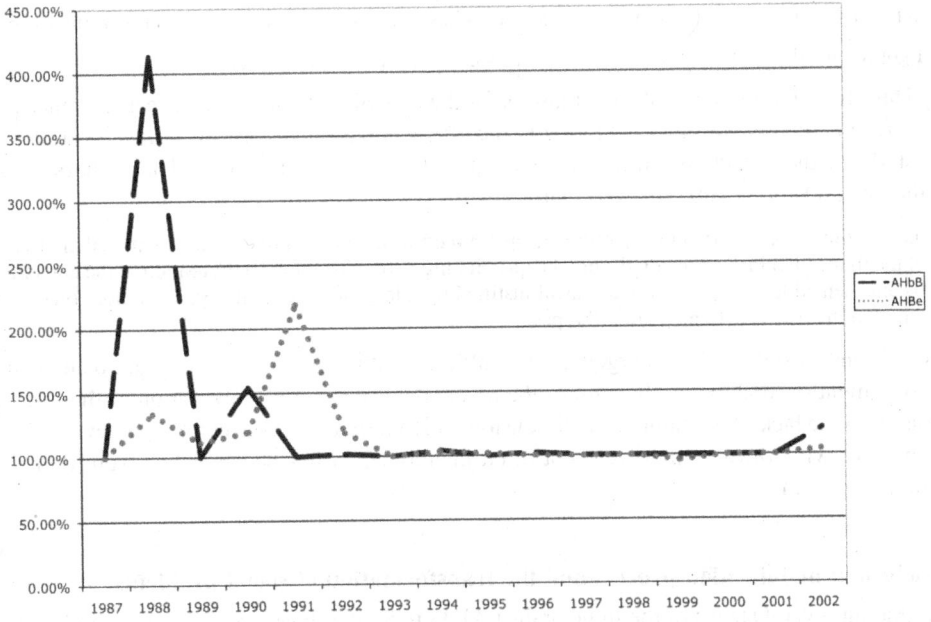

Figure 3. Evolution of public financing (in percentage terms) in comparison to the previous year (1987–2002).

From this perspective, participation would be both more limited over time and would involve individuals with a weaker link to the illness than in the earlier phase. This hypothesis could be supported by the indication that, for all those studied, there is a noticeable decline in affective proximity to the epidemic. Those who claimed that they had no acquaintances with HIV/AIDS rose from 32% between 1991 and 1996 to 40% between 1997 and 2001. This hypothesis is also supported by the fact that the withdrawal of the original activists in this phase marked the end of a long-standing involvement at a time when the fight against AIDS was being redefined and the motives for joining were changing (for an analysis of motives, cf. Fillieule 2001), making continuous involvement now more difficult.

Of the 27 respondents leaving anti-AIDS associations in the period 1996–2001, half did so in 2000. Heterosexual women represented most of those leaving (21 cases); eleven of them left the associative environment in 2000. Amongst those, seven left one of the cantonal associations that year. This defection was due to different motives. On one hand, for some the disengagement was related to the changing nature of participation within the collective, with a series of working groups disappearing during this period. On the other hand, and this is the reason for most of the withdrawals, those disengaging referred to motives related to the transformation of 'biographical availability' (Fillieule and Broqua 2005), in other words involvement and investment in competing social subsets. We find two illustrations of this below, the first reason for disengagement being offered by a woman involved since 1995, the second by a volunteer active since 1993. In the latter case, the reasons for withdrawal also relate to the difficulty of persisting in one's involvement following the upheaval provoked by the death of a person they were caring for:

> I have rebuilt my family life. I am happy to still have two children, so I am short of time.

> Return to studies and less time available. Last person cared for died.

Finally, a third type of motive is similar to that of biographical availability, but relates this issue to a feeling of exhaustion and of weariness in the area of HIV/AIDS. This is the case in the two following responses, the former involved since 1996 and the latter since 1991:

> When my husband and I had our son, we decided to take a breather. Fed up with HIV 100% of the time.

> I got involved in politics, and I felt a certain weariness, a need for a change.

Thus, for all of these people, the reasons for the defection do not make direct reference to the new therapeutic breakthrough but rather to the effects it has. Here, one may draw a parallel with the study of the defection within the Act Up and AIDES associations. The authors stressed (Fillieule and Broqua 2005, p. 200) that

> the most massive observable departures from 1996 on were only minimally due to the lethal effects of the illness, but instead resulted from the questioning born of the new configuration of the epidemic which seemed to encourage a withdrawal justified by a lack of availability or, even more often, by more conflictive situations than in the past.

The reasons linked to the emergence of conflictive situations did not appear to include the motives mentioned above in the case of the association. Instead, this evolution of the discourse is based on the lack of availability, a dimension which largely takes account of a new register of motives for withdrawal which were not often mentioned earlier because they were things that could not be said.

Conclusion: mobilization process and the transformation of social problems

In retracing several stages of the fight against AIDS in Switzerland, we wanted to emphasize the fact that, as Sawicki and Siméant (2009, p. 115) mentioned, 'activist organizations, *as organizations* and regardless of their degree of institutionalization, transform the individuals and are transformed by them'. It is important to remain attentive to factors contributing to shaping the mobilization starting first with the structuring of the homosexual associative space, then linking the resulting mobilization to the formation of the fight against AIDS, and finally detailing the various aspects of the transformation of the cause and the progressive institutionalization of the movement against the epidemic. Such an analysis remains attentive to the transformation of AIDS; examining the context of mobilization; and, finally, of linking the development and transformation of the AIDS cause to the evolution of the social characteristics of the actors who become involved, as well as to their reasons for engaging in the fight against the epidemic.

Examination of the development of the AIDS cause over a long period allows us to better understand how both a public policy, and social movement organizations, could become institutionalized at the same time, which decompartmentalizes questions too often examined separately (see Meyer 2005, Fillieule and Blanchard 2012 on this point). We argued here for an analysis of the development and transformation of causes as situated and contextualized, an analysis of the process of mobilization, careful to accurately depict those social actors who were the protagonists at the time and those who now are.

Over the course of this story, between the beginnings of the mobilization against the epidemic, when the urgency of taking action was paramount, and in its most recent developments, the AIDS cause has changed considerably. The current phase is characterized by attempts to diversify the fight. Nonetheless, there remains a profound indecisiveness following the 'normalization' of the cause, which led tangentially to treating AIDS as a social-health problem 'like any other'. In a context of budget cuts and trivialization of the epidemic, the cause is certainly at a turning point. Will we be witnessing the failure of a great cause to diversify, which Pollak (1990) described in another context or a success, at least temporarily, in repositioning the fight against AIDS consistent with the diversification of the issues and the objectives of mobilization?

Acknowledgements

We would like to thank Kent Buse and Dennis Altman, the editors of the present issue, as well as the reviewers for their valuable comments.

Notes

1. The concept of configuration is key to Elias' sociology of civilization. He defines these configurations as the changing pattern, which players form with each other, relations of suspense, interdependence of players *and* the fluctuating balance of suspense, the to-and-fro of a balance of power (Elias 1939).
2. The study combined archival analysis (reports and minutes produced by the voluntary groups, documents published by the Parliament as well as by the Federal Office of Public Health (FOPH) over the period), semi-structured interviews with activists of the Swiss Aids Federation, local AIDS groups, and members of the FOPH ($n = 41$), in depth interviews with activists ($n = 60$) and a quantitative analysis via a self-administered questionnaire sent to volunteers and ex-volunteers of eight associations during the Summer of 2005 ($n = 363$, answer rate 20.2%.) The study (dir., O. Fillieule, with M. Voegtli, S. Horat and P. Blanchard) was funded by the Swiss Scientific Funds 'Changes in AIDS epidemic, associational dynamics and commitment. Case Studies on seven swiss cantons' (3346C0-104177/1). See Voegtli (2009) for a detailed presentation of data and methods used.

References

Altman, D., 1994. *Power and community. Organizational and cultural responses to AIDS*. London: Taylor & Francis.

Armstrong, E.A., 2002. *Forging gay identities*. Chicago: University of Chicago Press.

Blumer, H., 1951 (1939. Collective behavior. *In*: A. McClung Lee, ed. *Principles of sociology*. New York: Barnes & Noble, 165–222.

Broqua, C., 2005. *Agir pour ne pas mourir. Act Up, les homosexuels et le sida*. Paris: Presses de Sciences Po.

Duyvendak, J.W., 1995. Gay subcultures between movement and market. *In*: H. Kriesi, ed. *New social movements in Western Europe. A comparative analysis*. London: University College London Press, 165–180.

Elias, N., 1939. *Über den Prozess der Zivilisation. Soziogenetische und psychogenetische Untersuchungen*. Frankfurt: Suhrkamp.

Elias, N., 1970. *Was ist Soziologie?* München: Juventa.

FF, 1996, 19th November. Message concernant une nouvelle loi sur l'organisation du gouvernement et de l'administration (LOGA) du 16 octobre 1996. *Feuille fédérale*, 5 (46) 1–23.

Fillieule, O., 2001. Propositions pour une analyse processuelle de l'engagement individuel. *Revue française de science politique*, 51 (1–2), 199–215.

Fillieule, O., 2010. Some elements of an interactionist approach to political disengagement. *Social Movement Studies*, 9 (1), 1–15.

Fillieule, O. and Blanchard, P., 2012. Fighting together. Assessing continuity and change in social movement organizations through the study of constituencies' heterogeneity. *In*: N. Kauppi, ed. *The new European political sociology*. Oxford: Routledge, 112–135.

Fillieule, O. and Broqua, C., 2005. La défection dans deux associations de lutte contre le sida: Act Up et AIDES. *In*: O. Fillieule, ed. *Le désengagement militant*. Paris: Belin, 189–228.

Giauque, D., 2003. New public management and organizational regulation: the liberal bureaucracy. *International Review of Administrative Sciences*, 69 (4), 567–592.

Herzlich, C., 2002. Vingt ans après ... l'évolution d'une épidémie. *Etudes*, 396 (2), 185–196.

Kippax, S., et al., 1993. *Sustaining safe sex. Gay communities respond to AIDS*. London: Falmer Press.

Kirp, D.L. and Bayer, R., 1992. The second decade of AIDS: the end of exceptionalism? *In*: D.L. Kirp and R. Bayer, eds. *AIDS in industrialized democracies. Passions, politics and policies*. Montréal: McGill–Queen's University Press, 361–384.

Kübler, D., et al., 2002. *Aidspolitik in der Schweiz: welche Normalisierung? Normalisierungsszenarien und Neue Partnerschaften in der HIV/Aidsprävention auf Bundesebene und in fuenf Kantonen*. Lausanne: Institut universitaire de médecine sociale et préventive.

Mellini, L., et al., 2004. *Le sida ne se dit pas. Analyse des formes de secret autour du VIH/sida*. Paris: L'Harmattan.

Meyer, D., 2005. Introduction. Social movements and public policy: eggs, chicken, and theory. *In*: D. Meyer et al., eds. *Routing the opposition. Social movements, public policy, and democracy*. Minneapolis: University of Minnesota Press, 1–26.

Pinell, P., et al., 2002. *Une épidémie politique. La lutte contre le sida en France 1981–1996*. Paris: PUF.

Pollak, M., 1988. *Les homosexuels et le sida: sociologie d'une épidémie*. Paris: Métailié.

Pollak, M., 1990. Constitution, diversification et échec de la généralisation d'une grande cause: le cas de la lutte contre le sida. *Politix*, 4 (16), 80–90.

Rosenbrock, R., et al., 2000. The normalization of AIDS in Western European countries. *Social Science and Medicine*, 50 (11), 1607–1629.

Sawicki, F. and Siméant, J., 2009. Décloisonner la sociologie de l'engagement militant. Note critique sur quelques tendances récentes des travaux français. *Sociologie du travail*, 51 (1), 97–125.

Schilling, R., 2000. The German AIDS self-help movement: the history and ongoing role of AIDS-Hilfe. *In*: R. Rosenbrock et al. eds. *Partnership and pragmatism. Germany's response to AIDS prevention and care*. London: Routledge, 82–90.

Setbon, M., 2000. La normalisation paradoxale du sida. *Revue française de sociologie*, 41 (1), 61–78.

Voegtli, M., 2009. *Emergence, constitution et diversification d'une cause. Processus de mobilisation, identités collectives et socialisations militantes dans l'espace associatif homosexuel et de lutte contre le sida en Suisse (1980–2005)*. Dissertation Thesis. Lausanne University and EHESS-Paris.

Whittier, N., 1997. Political generations, micro-cohorts, and the transformation of social movements. *American Sociological Review*, 62 (5), 760–778.

Wiltfang, G.L. and McAdam, D., 1991. The costs and risks of social activism: a study of sanctuary movement activism. *Social Forces*, 69 (4), 987–1010.

AIDS mobilisation in Zambia and Vietnam: explaining the differences

Amy S. Patterson and David Stephens

> This article compares AIDS mobilisation in Zambia and Vietnam. It looks specifically at the goals of AIDS movements in the two countries, arguing that the Vietnamese movement has been more singular in its focus with its major objective being to achieve representation of people living with HIV (PLHIVs) in AIDS decision-making. In Zambia, the movement has had multiple agendas: human rights protection, biomedical interventions, and economic development for PLHIVs. Instead of assessing how well the two movements have met these goals, the authors use insights from the scholarship on AIDS mobilisation to analyse why these different objectives exist. They argue that epidemic type, movement identity, political culture, and economic, political, and external structures lead to this variation. Through its cross-regional examination of significantly different countries, this comparative case study contributes to knowledge of AIDS mobilisation.

This article compares AIDS mobilisation in Vietnam and Zambia. It defines mobilisation as the organised efforts of non-state actors to influence state and donor policies and programmes on HIV and AIDS. The work looks specifically at the goals of AIDS mobilisation in the two countries, arguing that Vietnam's movement has had a more singular focus than Zambia's movement. While people living with HIV (PLHIVs) in Vietnam have been concerned about HIV prevention and human rights protection, they have prioritised gaining representation of PLHIVs in policymaking. In Zambia, the movement has had multiple agendas: urging adherence to antiretroviral treatment (ART), HIV prevention, and HIV testing; protecting human rights; and promoting economic development for PLHIVs. Our objective is not to assess how well the two movements have met these goals, but to explain why these goals differ. We use insights from the scholarship on AIDS mobilisation to argue that epidemic type, movement identity, political culture, and economic, political, and external structures led to this variation. Through its examination of significantly different countries, this comparative case study contributes to knowledge on AIDS mobilisation.

Lessons on AIDS mobilisation

The first factor that affects AIDS movements is the disease itself. The unusually high levels of suffering, loss, and stigma associated with AIDS drove participation in the USA (Jennings and Anderson 2003). But because every country has a unique AIDS epidemic based on its HIV prevalence rate and those populations at highest risk of infection, this epidemic variation may lead to differences in mobilisation. While countries with generalised epidemics (i.e. with national HIV rates above 1%) may have greater opportunities for broad-based mobilisation, the free rider problem may limit widespread participation and, if mobilisation occurs, large movements may become fragmented (de Waal 2006). In contrast, activism may be easier in countries with concentrated epidemics (i.e. national HIV rates below 1% and predominantly centred on specific populations at higher risk). In Malaysia and Singapore, for example, HIV has been mainly limited to sex workers, injecting drug users (IDUs), and transgender populations who have successfully mobilised (Weiss 2006). The length of time a country has experienced AIDS also may shape mobilisation, since some long-standing PLHIV organisations have become professional while others have become divided (Siplon 2002).

A second driver of mobilisation is a collective identity, which is a shared sense of 'we-ness' that leads to solidarity in and commitment to activism (Snow 2001). Identity is rooted in individuals' shifting subjectivities and personal experiences with AIDS (Robins 2006, p. 319). Identity can drive participation, as was the case for gay activists in the USA and Brazil, sex workers in India, and religious leaders concerned about HIV prevention in Brazil (Siplon 2002, Mello e Souza 2007, Ghose *et al.* 2008, Garcia and Parker 2011). But movement participation also can shape identity. In Singapore and Malaysia, participation in PLHIV movements contributed to a 'refinement' of activists' identity (Weiss 2006, p. 671). Mobilisation led activists in South Africa and Mozambique to emphasise civic ties in community relations, not their ethnic or religious identities (Fenio 2011, p. 730).

Third, as social movements are increasingly analysed outside of post-industrial societies, scholars recognise that political, historical, and cultural contexts condition AIDS mobilisation (Altman 1994, p. 157). The Treatment Action Campaign's historic roots in the antiapartheid movement taught its participants strategic communication and organisational skills (Johnson 2004). In North Africa, cultural patterns of patriarchy and anti-homosexual attitudes have shaped AIDS mobilisation (Roudi-Fahimi 2007), while in Senegal, culturally defined relations between Muslim leaders and their followers enabled those leaders to urge HIV prevention (Murphy 2004).

Finally, the social movement literature highlights the ways that opportunity structures, or political transformations, economic transitions, and access to global resources can shape mobilisation (Tilly 1978). In the late 1980s, AIDS activists capitalised on the fact that Brazil had transitioned to democracy and some state officials were from the gay, lesbian, and feminist movements and thus were sympathetic to AIDS activists (Headley and Siplon 2006). The success of The AIDS Support Organisation was partly due to the fact that it emerged just as Uganda's political system was stabilising after years of civil war and authoritarian rule (Muriisa 2010). Access to donor funding helped Brazilian religious leaders develop an effective AIDS advocacy network (Garcia and Parker 2011), and similar external ties enabled Indian PLHIV organisations to advocate for state funding for HIV programmes (Sridhar and Gómez 2011). But external linkages may also cause PLHIV groups to reconfigure their agendas to meet external demands or to reshape relations within their groups. In Tanzania, for example, local PLHIV groups' dependence on donors has led to factionalism and infighting, thus preventing activism (Beckman and Bujra 2010). To build ties to donors, PLHIV groups in Côte d'Ivoire urged members to disclose their HIV status, even though disclosure negatively affected individuals' relations with their family members (Nguyen 2010).

Country cases and methodology

Unlike single case studies, comparative case studies allow scholars to investigate how system-level traits affect outcomes (Manheim *et al.* 2008). While there have been some comparative studies of AIDS mobilisation (Headley and Siplon 2006, Weiss 2006, Fenio 2011, Patterson

2011), these studies have utilised cases within the same geographic regions, where countries are relatively similar in epidemic type, cultural patterns, governance structures, economic development, and relations with external actors. In contrast, we choose countries in different regions in order to isolate how our four variables affect AIDS movements. This work contributes to an emerging literature on cross-regional AIDS mobilisation (see Eboko *et al.* 2011).

Zambia and Vietnam provide several contrasts. First, their epidemics differ greatly, with HIV in Vietnam being concentrated primarily among IDUs, sex workers, and men who have sex with men (MSM), with HIV prevalence among these groups ranging from 3% to 50% (National Institute of Hygiene and Epidemiology & Vietnam Administration for HIV Prevention and Control 2009). In comparison, Zambia faces a generalised epidemic, with an HIV rate of approximately 14% among 15–49-year olds (Ministry of Health *et al.* 2010). Second, they differ in historical and cultural experiences. Zambia experienced mass mobilisation for independence in 1964 and multiparty democracy in 1990, but unlike Vietnam, its anticolonial struggle did not involve country division, an almost 20-year civil war that killed at least one million people, and violent occupation by foreign troops. Culturally, almost 85% of Zambians call themselves Christian, but the country has 73 official ethnic groups, many with their own language. Vietnam is nominally a Buddhist majority but with strong Confucian influence, and the Vietnamese population is relatively homogenous, with the Kinh (Viet) compiling roughly 86% of the population (Central Intelligence Agency (CIA) 2011).

In terms of structural variables, Zambia is a more democratic and free country than Vietnam. Despite centralised executive power and widespread corruption, Zambia protects many civil liberties and has a competitive political system (Freedom House 2010b). As a single-party state, Vietnam curtails political competition and limits freedom of the press, speech, religion, and association (Freedom House 2010a). While each country is poor, Vietnam's GDP per capita ($3000) is twice that of Zambia's ($1500). Vietnam has a growing industrial sector and export-oriented market which has fuelled urbanisation, while Zambia's economy relies heavily on copper exports and agriculture. Official development assistance comprised about 5% of Vietnam's GDP in 2009, compared to roughly 27% of Zambia's GDP (United Nations Development Programme (UNDP) 2010). Both countries have received donor funds for HIV/AIDS, though Zambia has received substantially more than Vietnam.

Despite these differences, PLHIV groups in both countries have participated in transnational AIDS movements. These movements have helped local PLHIV groups to build local capacity, recruit and train leaders, and articulate demands to government for ART access and anti-discrimination laws (Smith and Siplon 2006). In both Zambia and Vietnam, transnational movements have emphasised the Greater Involvement of People with AIDS (GIPA) initiative, which asserts that PLHIVs must be equal participants in all decision making on HIV and AIDS (see International HIV/AIDS Alliance 2008). Because PLHIV groups in both countries have these transnational linkages and because our goal is to examine how country differences shape PLHIV mobilisation, we do not include transnational linkages in our analysis.

To collect data, we conducted interviews and participant observations. Research focused on urban-based PLHIV groups, though these associations often had links to rural communities. The Zambian research was conducted in 2007 and 2011, while the Vietnamese fieldwork was conducted between 2002 and 2008. In order to ensure the comparability of data, one of the authors conducted additional interviews in Vietnam in 2011.

We used purposive sampling in order to choose interviewees representative of each country's AIDS movement. Because the Zambia movement has included both faith-based and secular groups, leaders and members of both types of PLHIV organisations were interviewed. Just as scholars assert that multiple organisations and actors comprise social movements (Snow 2001), we see Zambia's many PLHIV groups to be part of a singular movement intent on responding to AIDS. Secular groups were associated with the Network for Zambian People Living with HIV/AIDS (NZP+), while faith-based groups were aligned with Protestant and Catholic churches, the Zambia Network of Religious Leaders Living with or Personally Affected by HIV and AIDS (ZANERELA+), and the Zambian Interfaith Networking Group on HIV/AIDS (ZINGO). In Vietnam, leaders and members of the Bright Futures Group, the Vietnam National Network of People Living with HIV/AIDS (VNP+), and the Vietnam Positive Women's Network (VPWN) were interviewed. In order to triangulate the findings from the PLHIV groups, both authors interviewed donor and NGO representatives who worked with the PLHIV groups. Interviewees were asked about group history, activities, and relations with donors and the state; factors that shaped mobilisation; and challenges the groups faced. Seventy interviews were conducted in Zambia, and over 50 informal and formal interviews were done in Vietnam. All interviewees were assured they would remain anonymous.

Different movements and different goals

In the last decade, both Vietnam and Zambia have experienced growth in the number of non-state PLHIV organisations. In Zambia, the major PLHIV group – NZP+ – has established chapters in the country's 72 districts and many faith-based PLHIV organisations have formed. Both NZP+ and faith-based groups are represented on the National AIDS Council. As a result of mobilisation, the government agreed to provide free ART medications to those who qualify in 2005. However, after the government committed to this goal, the movement became disjointed with at least three discernible emphases (ZANERELA+ official, 30 March 2011).

The first goal is biomedical: HIV testing, ART adherence programmes for PLHIVs on treatment, and HIV prevention (Ministry of Health *et al.* 2010). PLHIV groups participate in these activities through community testing campaigns, adherence counselling, and grassroots AIDS education programmes. A second goal is the promotion of human rights and non-discrimination; some interviewees emphasised that, as a space where members could 'feel free' about their HIV status, PLHIV organisations reduce self-stigma, stand against discrimination, and promote PLHIV participation in community decision making (NZP+ leaders, 18 April 2011 and 7 March 2011, ZINGO official, 17 August 2007, Church AIDS official, 10 March 2011). The third goal is fostering development through income-generating activities, since the lack of food security, shelter, and education prevent PLHIVs from living positively (NZP+ leaders, 21 March 2011 and 4 July 2011, NZP+ member, 24 March 2011, Church PLHIV group member, 9 March 2011). To meet this goal, activists tended to target donors to provide funds for such projects, not government to meet the structural challenges of job creation or income inequality (NZP+ leader, 7 March 2011). According to a long-time AIDS policy observer in Zambia, the lack of common goals among PLHIVs made mobilisation difficult (1 May 2011).

In contrast, Vietnam's movement became more unified since its inception and despite its growth. From its origins as a small group of PLHIVs in Hanoi, the movement now comprises two national networks, VNP+ and VPWN, several regional and provincial networks, and over 200 local groups. While the movement now engages in several activities that Zambian groups do, PLHIVs play a very limited role in AIDS counselling and support programmes. The movement retains a strong focus on working with and convincing policymakers that PLHIVs can and should have a larger role than merely peer education in HIV programme and policy responses, since much AIDS policymaking has been 'top-down', not 'bottom-up' (Ha *et al.* 2010). These groups want government to recognise their legitimate and viable role as representatives of communities living with and affected by AIDS. While VNP+ gained representation on key national committees in 2009, and senior government and party members court PLHIVs for events such as World AIDS Day, the goal of PLHIV representation has not been fully met. The movement wants increased representation of provincial and local groups in a national PLHIV advocacy agenda, and it demands authentic representation not mere tokenism (PLHIV, 9 September 2011).

Explaining differences in mobilisation

While there is some overlap between Vietnamese and Zambian PLHIV movements, each movement's unity and the breadth of its agenda differ. We turn to lessons from the literature on AIDS mobilisation to analyse these contrasts. In so doing, we do not prioritise one explanation over others.

Two different epidemics

Although it took Zambian PLHIV groups a decade to form after the country's first AIDS case appeared in 1984, PLHIV groups have a longer history than Vietnamese groups because the epidemic first emerged in southern Africa (Ministry of Health *et al.* 2010). While NZP+ formed in 1996, most faith-based groups started around 2000, a fact that has led to divisions in mobilisation. Because of the country's high HIV rate and its almost 30-year history with AIDS, the disease has affected many Zambians (Afrobarometer 2004), and the PLHIV movement has the potential to be quite large. The population's experiences with the disease have led to a decline in stigma (Nyblade *et al.* 2003), with some respondents claiming in 2011 that stigma was 'no longer a problem' (ZANERELA+ official, 30 March 2011, NZP+ member, 24 March 2011). Additionally, women comprise about 60% of PLHIVs. Even though they dominate PLHIV groups, their marginalisation in society makes it more difficult for them to lead a unified movement (Ministry of Health *et al.* 2010, NZP+ leader, 21 March 2011).The disease's broad effect on society, the decline in stigma, the different histories of PLHIV groups, and women's predominant role as group members complicate PLHIV mobilisation around a unified agenda (AIDS expert, 1 May 2011).

As in Zambia, it took PLHIV groups in Vietnam roughly a decade to organise after the first reported HIV infection in 1990. In the face of state repression, the first PLHIV groups began in 2002, eight years after NZP+ started. Concentrated in IDUs, female sex workers, and MSM, Vietnam's epidemic touches the most marginalised people in society. Even though gender inequality is a barrier in the AIDS response in both countries (Wischermann 2010), it has a different effect in Vietnam since 70% of people infected with HIV are men and male PLHIV group leaders have not faced gender-based social and political marginalisation (Government of Vietnam 2010). While the epidemic's smaller scale, concentrated nature, and shorter history could potentially hamper mobilisation, these factors have necessitated that PLHIVs build a unified agenda. In fact, today VNP+ is arguably the most successful national PLHIV network in the Asia and Pacific region (Paxton and Janssen 2009). In sum, the countries' different epidemics shape movement unity and agenda setting.

Competing or collective identities?

PLHIV identity contrasts in each country's movement. While many Zambian PLHIVs acknowledge shared experiences with HIV, differences in religion, gender, income, education, age, and even sero-status (if mobilisation includes HIV-negative caregivers) hamper unity. Here we focus on the contrasting ways faith-based and secular groups defined identity. Because NZP+ was rooted in the GIPA principles, NZP+ groups only contained PLHIVs as members (NZP+ leader, 4 July 2011). In contrast, faith-based groups often included co-religionists affected by HIV, many of whom served as caregivers; these groups rooted identity not in sero-status but in religious affiliation (ZANERELA+ official, 30 March 2011). While caregivers' involvement often reflected their religious beliefs about service, some caregivers had not been tested for HIV, a fact that showed their ambivalence about an HIV-related identity (Church AIDS official, 25 February 2011).

These two identities – HIV positivity in NZP+ groups and religious identity in faith-based groups – made it difficult to forge more than ad hoc collaboration across these two organisational types. A pattern of inter-group competition emerged, particularly in urban neighbourhoods, where it was not unusual for several PLHIV groups to exist and for community members to move between them depending on the groups' programmes. Competing groups rarely pooled resources for joint training sessions, voluntary counselling and testing efforts, or World AIDS Day events. Group agendas varied: NZP+ stressed stigma reduction and poverty alleviation, while faith-based groups emphasised care and HIV prevention (Church PLHIV member, 21 May 2011, NZP+ leader, 21 March 2011).

In Vietnam, PLHIV groups have worked to forge a shared identity, which has then made it possible to agree on the goal of representation and to work toward that goal. From the early days of PLHIV mobilisation, the key challenge of creating an organising identity has been the stigma of HIV. During the 1990s and the early years of the new millennium, Vietnamese AIDS policy linked HIV with the 'moral contagion' of sex work and illicit drug use. Public HIV information campaigns depicted images of wasting and dying people with AIDS, whom the government asserted had been overcome by these 'evils' (Ha *et al.* 2010). One PLHIV explained the effect of this environment: 'It was a difficult thing for me to disclose that I was HIV positive. I did, but many others felt they could not. There was so much fear and stigma' (PLHIV, 9 September 2011). The belief among government officials and health-care providers that PLHIVs could not contribute to the country's AIDS response also increased stigma: 'People in power had no recognition or idea about the value of or role of a PLHIV group or network.... It was not possible to think of PLHIVs as anything more than weak and stigmatised' (NGO member, 7 September 2011). It was necessary to develop a collective identity to combat these views.

Despite stigma, discrimination, and fear, small groups of PLHIVs did emerge around 2000 to support their members and their members' families. These groups became a foundation on which larger PLHIV networks were built. As these networks emerged, they had to come to terms with externally imposed stigma. To distance themselves from drug use and sex work and to develop their own identity, some groups imposed rules which required members and/or leaders to pledge that they did not currently inject drugs or engage in sex work (PLHIV group observation, 14 April 2004). This strategy, however, did not contribute to a broader HIV identity that crossed lines of sexuality or behavioural practices.

A more inclusive collective identity emerged between 2004 and 2005 as groups began to engage with the government and international agencies on HIV education and advocacy. PLHIV organisations assessed which marginalised identity (HIV status, on the one hand, or drug use and sex work, on the other) would be acceptable in national and local political processes. They delinked HIV from drug use and sex work in their rhetoric, creating a collective identity that downplayed underlying issues of behaviour and sexuality. This helped to mobilise PLHIVs for participation in policymaking and service delivery. Collective identity formation was possible because several founders of the PLHIV movement have a background in drug use and understand the issues this population faces (PLHIV, 9 September 2011). Yet, even though this broad HIV identity has benefited the movement, one PLHIV group member (7 September 2011) cautioned that in the long term, it may make it harder to advocate against the legal and policy barriers that directly affect IDUs and sex workers.

Political culture: patronage networks of dependence versus collective self-reliance

While patronage networks, dependence on external assistance, and collective values exist in both countries, patronage and dependence are more pronounced in Zambia and collectivism is more evident in Vietnam. In Zambia, ethnic ties affect voting behaviour and shape access to state resources and economic opportunities. Patronage networks dominate society, and lower status individuals turn to ethnic or religious leaders to access material resources in return for loyalty (Posner 2005). These particularistic ties affected PLHIV groups (see Beckman and Bujra 2010). The existence of so many faith-based and NZP+ groups partly reflects local patrons' desire to build a following and to reward followers with resources, many of which come from donors (NGO official, 31 March 2011). This pattern was also rooted in the churches' historic role in politics and service delivery (Patterson 2011). But instead of a unified faith-based PLHIV group, specific churches have formed their own organisations, further dividing the movement (ZANERELA+ official, 30 March 2011, ZINGO official, 17 August 2007).

Patronage expectations also affected ties between leaders and followers in PLHIV groups. Because donors worked closely with caregivers, these individuals often became group leaders and had access to material goods that rank-in-file members wanted. This practice was evident in the vast majority of the 57 PLHIV groups observed. According to interviewees, caregivers became patrons in their organisations, building a following of loyal 'clients'. (Church AIDS official, 25 February 2011, AIDS clinic social worker, 31 March 2011) These patron–client relations could hamper group unity: some members said that caregivers did not always give clients resources, preferring to share them with family instead. Since clients depended on these caregivers for assistance, they rarely protested (Church PLHIV group member, 7 April 2011, NZP+ leader, 15 April 2011). Patronage interacted with Zambia's history of foreign aid dependence since the 1960s, a phenomenon that some scholars claim has created a culture of dependence (Moyo 2009). Access to foreign aid became a patronage tool, though it limited group self-reliance. As one NZP+ leader said, 'We have to learn to get up and do for ourselves, not to wait for others to come help us' (18 April 2011).

Collectivism, or the maintenance of positive relations within the community and high levels of group cooperation, is a central value in Vietnam (Parks and Vu 1994). Vietnamese civil society groups, including PLHIV groups, emphasise respect and compromise (Wischermann 2010). The country's long nationalist struggle against French colonialism and American occupation also contributed to a sense of national identity and self-reliance, as did the country's international isolation between roughly 1975 and 1990. While no interviewee explicitly said these values determined PLHIV movement unity, because these cultural traits have affected other civil society groups, we believe they influence PLHIV organisations. Unlike Zambia, because organised religion plays a minor role in Vietnam, faith-based groups did not form large-scale PLHIV groups. Thus, Vietnam's political culture contributed to a singular PLHIV agenda, while patronage networks, particularistic ties, religious organisations, and donor dependence hampered this unity in Zambia.

Economic, political, and external structures

Zambia's pervasive poverty drives some PLHIV organisations to focus on poverty-reduction programmes that stretch beyond HIV and AIDS per se. The need for income-generation has become even more pronounced with the introduction of free ART: 'Having free ARVs does not do any good if people don't have enough to eat. They can't take the drugs because they get sick. Then they stop taking their medicines. How does that fight AIDS?' (NZP+ member, 27 June 2011). Yet the poverty-reduction agenda competes with the human rights and biomedical agendas if PLHIV groups merely become 'projects' that ignore stigma reduction or gender vulnerability (NZP+ leader, 7 March 2011). Poverty makes individuals rely on local patrons and donors for assistance, and it causes impoverished PLHIVs to emphasise their gender, religious, and/or HIV identities to access resources, particularly food. In contrast, because Vietnam's epidemic is concentrated, AIDS programmes have not typically extended into a broader development framework. While HIV has a negative effect on PLHIVs and their families, the country's Comprehensive Poverty Reduction and Growth Strategy does not consider HIV to be a development issue (Government of Vietnam 2003). Thus, poverty reduction has not become a competing agenda item for PLHIV groups.

In terms of politics, Zambia's democratic transition in the 1990s widened the political space for civil society activity and urged the involvement of faith-based and community-based organisations in local development activities. At times, organisations (including PLHIV groups) have competed for finite resources and political influence. Competition and disorganisation among PLHIV groups has meant that they do not all have an equal voice in policymaking, with faith-based groups that support HIV prevention and service delivery having more influence than NZP+ groups that urge human rights protection (Donor official, 23 February 2011, Church AIDS official, 20 August 2007, Kelly and Birdsall 2010).

Even though the Vietnamese state has allowed non-state affiliated groups to exist in recent years (Wells-Dang 2010), civil society is quite underdeveloped. Vietnam's complex legal framework limits associational autonomy. For example, while the 2006 HIV law encourages faith-based and non-governmental organisations to participate in the AIDS response, no Vietnamese legal document explicitly authorises the existence of civil society organisations (Hammett *et al.* 2011). Even though government relies on NGOs to meet some AIDS service demands, many of these NGOs are extensions of the state, and thus they do not challenge state policies on human rights (Thayer 2009). The state ideology that the 'Party knows best' and the state's suspicion of an independent civil society have been evident as PLHIV groups have sought representation (Sidel 2010). One NGO staff member (8 September 2011) explained:

> Government at first did not accept these ideas [of PLHIV representation]. There was very deep discrimination towards PLHIVs. The attitude being, 'How can these people do anything useful? They are only good at taking drugs'. I remember the first meetings where we brought PLHIV and government officials together in 2003 and it was a revelation to the officials, who until that time had never knowingly met a person with HIV.

The difficult political environment has required Vietnamese PLHIV groups to be more unified in their objectives than Zambian groups.

State policy agendas may provide moments for mobilisation or demobilisation. Zambia's adoption of a free ART policy in 2005 deflated energy from the AIDS movement, since secular and faith-based activists subsequently lacked a singular galvanising issue (NZP+ leader, 19 May 2011, Church AIDS official, 9 May 2011). In contrast, the Vietnamese government's acceptance of harm reduction approaches in 2006, including needle and syringe distribution and methadone maintenance therapy, provided a new space in which IDUs and the NGOs working with them could organise. These policy changes were 'not characterized by intensive discussions in society', but rather reflected greater political commitment and access to accurate HIV information among Communist Party leaders (Ha *et al.* 2010, p. 8). While IDUs are still subject to arrest and confinement in drug rehabilitation centres, harm reduction has allowed IDUs to develop their own groups and to build ties to broader PLHIV networks (Reid and Higgs 2011). The policy change provided an opportunity to create a collective PLHIV identity and then to demand representation.

Access to donor resources also affected mobilisation. As of 2006, donors funded roughly 77% of Zambia's AIDS response; between 2003 and 2010, the country had received 13 HIV-related grants from The Global Fund to Fight AIDS, Tuberculosis and Malaria (the Global Fund) and almost one billion dollars from the US Emergency Plan for AIDS Relief (PEPFAR) (Ministry of Health *et al.* 2010, PEPFAR 2010a, Global Fund to Fight AIDS,

Tuberculosis and Malaria 2011b). Similarly, external donors funded between 80% and 90% of the Vietnamese AIDS response in 2006 (Martinez 2008). Between 2003 and 2010, Vietnam received four Global Fund HIV-related grants, and between 2006 and 2010, roughly $300 million from PEPFAR (PEPFAR 2010b, Global Fund to Fight AIDS, Tuberculosis and Malaria 2011a). In both countries, this influx of funding led to the growth of an NGO sector, eager to access donor funds (Vietnamese NGO official, 8 September 2011, Zambian NGO official, 31 March 2011). But this funding has affected each country differently.

In Zambia, donors spent roughly half of their resources on ART distribution and adherence, one-fourth on prevention, and only 4% on impact mitigation (Ministry of Health *et al.* 2010). The donor field was diverse and expansive, as indicated by the presence of a large number of international NGOs (see PEPFAR 2007b). Donor treatment programmes shaped community expectations about the benefits of PLHIV mobilisation, a pattern that emerged because of recipients' dependence on donors. From 2004 to 2008, donors provided food supplements to people who began ART and funding to newly formed PLHIV groups in order to facilitate the scale up of ART. During this period, many bilateral donors and international NGOs considered AIDS to be an 'emergency' that needed immediate responses such as HIV testing, ART access, and food distribution (NGO officials, 17 and 31 March 2011, NZP+ leader, 15 April 2011). As a result, many impoverished PLHIVs associated AIDS with access to material benefits: 'People just expected that the donors were going to bring them food if they were HIV-positive' (NGO official, 31 March 2011).

By 2011 almost 70% of Zambians who needed ART could access it. Donor programmes then sought to empower PLHIVs with income-generation projects and health education (NGO officials, 20 and 21 May 2011). Yet, when individuals joined PLHIV groups after 2008 they continued to expect material benefits. Home-based caregivers bemoaned their lack of resources to share (Caregiver, 20 May 2011). Without patronage to bind together people who had only their sero-status in common, group members quit (PLHIV, 2 March 2011, NZP+ members, 27 and 28 March 2011). Groups also increasingly competed for donor resources, and the more successful PLHIV groups emphasised their desperation, showcased their efforts, and downplayed the work of other PLHIV groups (NZP+ leader, 21 March 2011, Church PLHIV group member, 10 March 2011). These processes contributed to inter-group suspicion and hampered mobilisation (NZP+ leader, 18 March 2011).

Donors played a slightly different role in Vietnam. While they devoted one-third of resources to treatment and care, they emphasised HIV prevention and civil society empowerment more than in Zambia (Government of Vietnam 2010). Their approach reflects the neoliberal values of Vietnam's largest donor, the US government (through PEPFAR). These values stressed the need for an autonomous civil society to counter state power and provide services, and a belief that the Vietnamese government's portrayal of PLHIVs as 'social evils' encroached on the rights of PLHIVs and ultimately, harmed the AIDS response (Ha *et al.* 2010). In prevention, donors supported the dissemination of HIV information and harm reduction, the distribution of condoms, and the development of methadone maintenance programmes. They stressed individual autonomy and human rights protection, a public health approach that directly challenged the state's focus on harsh punishment for illegal behaviour and its emphasis on protecting the community over individuals (Giang and Huong 2009). The public health approach directly aligned with the goals of Vietnam's PLHIV movement (NGO member, 7 September 2011).

Donors also helped to create political space for PLHIV groups, by providing them with funding and logistical support as they began to directly dialogue with the Vietnamese government (see Thayer 2009). Donors' emphasis on the GIPA principles galvanised PLHIV groups to develop a common objective (Paxton and Janssen 2009). Donors brought together government and PLHIV representatives in several national-level consultations to draft the country's 2006

HIV law. This process further advanced PLHIV mobilisation as the leading groups sought the participation of the wider PLHIV population (Khuat 2007). In order to empower civil society, donors also have limited the funds they provide directly to the Vietnamese state, relying more on international NGOs and their local partners (including some PLHIV groups) for project implementation (see PEPFAR 2007a). These donor actions have helped to unify the PLHIV movement and to legitimate its demand for representation.

Conclusion

In summary, Zambia's broad-based epidemic has made collective identity formation difficult and challenged mobilisation, while Vietnam's concentrated epidemic has had the opposite effect. Particularistic ties, patronage networks, and the autonomous role of religion have complicated mobilisation in Zambia, while values of collectivism and self-reliance have urged agenda unity in Vietnam. Political pluralism and donor priorities in Zambia have created not only space for a PLHIV movement, but also the opportunity for greater divisions in the movement's agenda. In contrast, fighting for political space has been a goal of Vietnamese PLHIV groups (and their donor supporters) because of the authoritarian nature of the state. Donors have urged a human rights agenda and GIPA principles, a process that fostered a more collective HIV identity.

This work contributes new insights to the social movement literature, which has tended to emphasise how resources, social and cultural context, and political opportunities shape mobilisation, but has downplayed how epidemiological factors influence movements (Smith and Siplon 2006). The Zambia–Vietnam comparison highlights how differences in HIV rates, epidemic histories, and infected populations influence the development of a unified movement agenda. We also raise new questions about the ways donors' different priorities and socioeconomic and political structures interact to affect local mobilisation. The Zambia–Vietnam study shows that donors can have different objectives, with service delivery being the focus in Zambia and civil society empowerment emphasised in Vietnam. Yet because of poverty and patronage networks, donor agendas negatively influenced mobilisation in Zambia. In Vietnam, however, the country's narrow political space necessitated donor objectives to build civil society capacity. Given the decline in global funding for HIV (Kaiser Family Foundation 2011), questions about the fluidity of donor priorities and the effect of those priorities on PLHIV organisations and mobilisation must continue to be investigated.

Acknowledgements

The authors wish to thank the US Fulbright African Research Scholar Program and Calvin College for financial support, as well as Dennis Altman, Kent Buse, Corwin Smidt, and two reviewers for helpful suggestions.

References

Afrobarometer, 2004. *Public opinion and HIV/AIDS: facing up to the future?* Available from: http://www.afrobarometer.org/AfrobriefNo12.pdf [accessed 15 July 2005].

Altman, D., 1994. *Power and community: organizational and cultural responses to AIDS*. Abingdon: Taylor & Francis.

Beckman, N. and Bujra, J., 2010. The 'politics of the queue': the politicization of people living with HIV/AIDS in Tanzania. *Development and Change*, 41 (6), 1041–1064.

Central Intelligence Agency (CIA), 2011. *CIA world factbook*. Available from: https://www.cia.gov/library/publications/the-world-factbook/ [accessed 29 December 2011].

Eboko, F., Bourdier, F. and Broqua, C., 2011. *Les Suds face au sida. Quand le société civile se mobilise.* Marseille: IRD editions.

Fenio, K., 2011. Tactics of resistance and the evolution of identity from subjects to citizens: the AIDS political movement in Southern Africa. *International Studies Quarterly*, 55 (3), 717–735.

Freedom House, 2010a. *Country report Vietnam*. Available from: http://www.freedomhouse.org/template.cfm?page=22&country=7949&year=2010 [accessed 2 January 2012].

Freedom House, 2010b. *Country report Zambia*. Available from: http://freedomhouse.org/template.cfm?page=22&country=7951&year=2010 [accessed 2 January 2012].

Garcia, J. and Parker, R., 2011. Resource mobilization for health advocacy: Afro-Brazilian religious organizations and HIV prevention and control. *Social Science & Medicine*, 72 (12), 1930–1938.

Ghose, T., *et al.*, 2008. Mobilizing collective identity to reduce HIV risk among sex workers in Sonagachi, India: the boundaries, consciousness, negotiation framework. *Social Science & Medicine*, 67 (2), 311–320.

Giang, L.M. and Huong, N.T.M., 2009. New bottle, but old wine: from family planning to HIV/AIDS in post-Doi Moi Vietnam. *Global Public Health*, 3 (S2), 76–91.

Global Fund to Fight AIDS, Tuberculosis and Malaria, 2011a. *Grant Portfolio – Vietnam*. Available from: http://portfolio.theglobalfund.org/en/Country/Index/VTN/ [accessed 1 January 2012].

Global Fund to Fight AIDS, Tuberculosis and Malaria, 2011b. *Grant Portfolio-Zambia*. Available from: http://portfolio.theglobalfund.org/en/Grant/List/ZAM [accessed 1 January 2012].

Government of Vietnam, 2003. *Comprehensive poverty reduction and growth strategy*. Available from: http://siteresources.worldbank.org/INTVIETNAM/Overview/20270134/cprgs_finalreport_Nov03.pdf [accessed 17 October 2011].

Government of Vietnam, 2010. *Fourth country report on following up the implementation of the declaration of commitment on HIV and AIDS*. Available from: http://www.unaids.org/en/dataanalysis/monitoringcountryprogress/2010progressreportssubmittedbycountries/vietnam_2010_country_progress_report_en.pdf [accessed 26 December 2011].

Ha, P. *et al.*, 2010. The evolution of HIV policy in Vietnam: from punitive control measures to a more rights-based approach. *Global Health Action*, 3 (August). Available from: http://www.globalhealthaction.net/index.php/gha/article/view/4625 [accessed 20 September 2011].

Hammett, T.M., Tiedemann, M. and Khuat, T.H.O., 2011. *Policy brief: the role of civil society organizations in Vietnam's HIV/AIDS response*. Hanoi: USAID Health Policy Initiative Vietnam.

Headley, J. and Siplon, P., 2006. Roadblocks on the road to treatment: lessons from Barbados and Brazil. *Perspectives on Politics*, 4 (4), 655–661.

International HIV/AIDS Alliance, 2008. *Nothing about us without us*. Available from: http://www.aidsalliance.org/includes/Publication/Nothing_About_Us_REPORT_English.pdf [accessed 22 September 2011].

Jennings, M. and Anderson, E., 2003. The importance of social and political context: the case of AIDS activism. *Political Behavior*, 25 (2), 177–199.

Johnson, K., 2004. The politics of AIDS policy development and implementation in postapartheid South Africa. *Africa Today*, 51 (2), 107–128.

Kaiser Family Foundation, 2011. *Kaiser/UNAIDS study finds drop in overall disbursements for AIDS response in 2010, seven out of 15 governments report reductions*. [News release]. Available from: http://www.kff.org/hivaids/hiv081511nr.cfm [accessed 17 October 2011].

Kelly, K. and Birdsall, K., 2010. The effects of national and international HIV/AIDS funding and governance mechanisms on the development of civil-society responses to HIV/AIDS in East and Southern Africa. *AIDS Care*, 22 (2), 1580–1587.

Khuat, T.H.O., 2007. *HIV policy in Vietnam: a civil society perspective*. Report for Open Society Institute. Available from: http://www.soros.org/initiatives/health/focus/phw/articles_publications/publications/vietnam_20071129/vietnam_20071129.pdf [accessed 17 October 2011].

Manheim *et al.*, 2008. *Empirical political analysis*. New York: Pearson Longman.

Martinez, J., 2008. *How external support for health and HIV will evolve as Viet Nam becomes a middle-income country*. Report commissioned by the UN Country Team Vietnam. Available from: http://www.wpro.who.int/NR/rdonlyres/C2A5BD91-0CF8-4F07-9B72-B3D0E9FFED0E/0/mic_report.pdf [accessed 30 September 2011].

Mello e Souza, A., 2007. Defying globalization: effective self-reliance in Brazil. *In*: P. Harris and P. Siplon, eds. *The global politics of AIDS*. Boulder, CO: Lynne Rienner Publishers, 37–64.

Ministry of Health, National AIDS Council and UNAIDS, 2010. *Zambia country progress report. UNGASS 2010 reporting*. Available from: http://www.unaids.org/en/dataanalysis/monitoringcountryprogress/2010progressreportssubmittedbycountries/zambia_2010_country_progress_report_en.pdf [accessed 30 May 2011].

Moyo, D., 2009. *Dead aid: why aid is not working and why there is a better way for Africa.* New York: Farrar, Straus and Giroux.

Muriisa, R., 2010. The role of NGOs in addressing gender inequality and HIV/AIDS in Uganda. *Canadian Journal of African Studies*, 44 (3), 605–623.

Murphy, J., 2004. Senegal fights to stay ahead of HIV, AIDS. *Baltimore Sun*. Available from: http://articles.baltimoresun.com/2004-05-23/news/0405230178_1_senegal-infections-hiv [accessed 1 January 2012].

National Institute of Hygiene and Epidemiology & Vietnam Administration for HIV/AIDS Prevention and Control, 2009. *HIV/STI integrated behavioral and biological surveillance in Vietnam, round 2.* Hanoi: Ministry of Health.

Nguyen, V., 2010. *The republic of therapy: triage and sovereignty in West Africa's time of AIDS.* Chapel Hill, NC: Duke University Press.

Nyblade, L. et al., 2003. *Disentangling HIV and AIDS stigma in Ethiopia, Tanzania and Zambia.* Report for International Center for Research on Women. Available from: http://www.icrw.org/publications/disentangling-hiv-and-aids-stigma-ethiopia-tanzania-and-zambia [accessed 11 November 2009].

Parks, C. and Vu, A., 1994. Social dilemma behavior of individuals from highly individualist and collectivist cultures. *Journal of Conflict Resolution*, 38 (4), 708–718.

Patterson, A., 2011. *The church and AIDS in Africa: the politics of ambiguity.* Boulder, CO: First Forum Press.

Paxton, S. and Janssen, P.L., 2009. *AusAID GIPA scoping report.* Available from: http://www.ausaid.gov.au/keyaid/hivaids/pdfs/gipa-scoping-1209.pdf [accessed 18 October 2011].

Posner, D., 2005. *Institutions and ethnic politics in Africa.* New York: Cambridge Press.

President's Emergency Plan for AIDS Relief (PEPFAR), 2007a. *Vietnam partners.* Available from: http://www.pepfar.gov/countries/c19722.htm [accessed 27 December 2011].

President's Emergency Plan for AIDS Relief (PEPFAR), 2007b. *Zambia partners.* Available from: http://www.pepfar.gov/countries/c19725.htm [accessed 27 December 2011].

President's Emergency Plan for AIDS Relief (PEPFAR), 2010a. *Budget spending- Zambia.* Available from: http://www.pepfar.gov/about/2010/africa/150629.htm [accessed 17 September 2011].

President's Emergency Plan for AIDS Relief (PEPFAR), 2010b. *PEPFAR 2010 overview.* Available from: http://vietnam.usembassy.gov/pepfar.html [accessed 17 September 2011].

Reid, G. and Higgs, P., 2011. Vietnam moves forward with harm reduction: an assessment of progress. *Global Public Health*, 6 (2), 168–180.

Robins, S., 2006. From 'rights' to 'ritual': AIDS activism in South Africa. *American Anthropologist*, 108 (2), 312–323.

Roudi-Fahimi, F., 2007. *Time to intervene: preventing the spread of HIV/AIDS in the Middle East and North Africa.* Washington, DC: Population Reference Bureau.

Sidel, M., 2010. Maintaining firm control: recent developments in nonprofit law and regulation in Vietnam. *International Journal of Not-For-Profit Law*, 12 (3). Available from: http://ecbiz108.inmotionhosting.com~icnlor5/research/journal/vol12iss3/art_1.htm [accessed 22 September 2010].

Siplon, P., 2002. *AIDS and the policy struggle in the United States.* Washington, DC: Georgetown University Press.

Smith, R. and Siplon, P., 2006. *Drugs into bodies: global AIDS treatment activism.* Westport, CT: Praeger Publishers.

Snow, D., 2001. Collective identity and expressive forms. *In*: N.J. Smelser and P.B. Baltes, eds. *International encyclopaedia of the social and behavioural sciences*. London: Elsevier Science, 196–254.

Sridhar, D. and Gómez, E., 2011. Health financing in Brazil, Russia and India: what role does the international community play? *Health Politics and Planning*, 26 (1), 12–24.

Thayer, C.A., 2009. Vietnam and the challenge of political civil society. *Contemporary Southeast Asia: A Journal of International & Strategic Affairs*, 31 (1), 1–27.

Tilly, C., 1978. *From mobilization to revolution.* New York: Random House.

United Nations Development Programme (UNDP), 2010. *Human development report 2010.* Available from: http://www.beta.undp.org/content/dam/undp/library/corporate/HDR/HDR_2010_EN_Complete_reprint-1.pdf [accessed 22 September 2011].

de Waal, A., 2006. *AIDS and power: why there is no political crisis yet.* London: Zed Books.

Weiss, M., 2006. Rejection as freedom? HIV/AIDS organizations and identity. *Perspectives on Politics*, 4 (4), 671–678.

Wells-Dang, A., 2010. Political space in Vietnam: a view from the 'rice roots'. *The Pacific Review*, 23 (1), 93–112.

Wischermann, J., 2010. Civil society action and governance in Vietnam: selected findings from an empirical survey. *Journal of Current Southeast Asian Affairs*, 29 (2), 3–40.

China's evolving AIDS policy: the influence of global norms and transnational non-governmental organizations

Joan Kaufman

China is moving towards greater rule of law and more accountable governance, including civil society participation. China's AIDS response has moved from denial to pragmatic policy. This change has come both through global influence and domestic pressure and led to adoption of many international norms for prevention, treatment, and care, sometimes in conflict with cultural attitudes and political positions. Connections between China's AIDS non-governmental organizations (NGOs) and transnational civil society organizations have contributed to transfer of new norms and approaches. Policies on sex worker rights, NGOs' role in governance, legal protection from discrimination, compensation for some infected by medical procedures, and intellectual property rights for essential medicines have begun to change. Advocacy and expert input from domestic NGOs connected to global groups have played a role. This paper argues that these soft power processes accompanying globalization are creating inroads even in China regarding universal human rights and protection of citizen's interests.

Introduction

The power of transnational social movements to advance human rights and social justice on a variety of issues is a growing reality of our increasingly interconnected world. But country contexts and political realities have a major influence on how far these social movements can progress: the presence and strength of national civil society relative to government limits efforts that may be in conflict with national policies. There has been a sea change in China's response to its AIDS epidemic since the first case of AIDS was identified in 1985. China has moved from denial and inaction to a national policy based on many international best practices and universal principles of justice. This change has come about through a combination of global influence and domestic pressure, resulting in the transfer and adoption of internationally accepted norms and approaches for AIDS prevention, treatment and care, sometimes in conflict with cultural attitudes and political positions. China's emerging civil society actors and their connections with transnational civil society (TNCS) organizations working on key elements of the AIDS response has provided one important mechanism for this transfer of knowledge and approaches. Their efforts working with grassroots organizations and informal alliances, often in tandem with advocacy by global development institutions has instigated movement on a number of policy fronts.

In this article, I will examine several issues that have been influenced by TNCS organizing: HIV prevention for sex workers, non-governmental organization (NGO) representation on the Global Fund's country coordinating mechanism (CCM), protection from discrimination for people living with HIV, legal compensation for persons accidentally infected with HIV, and China's positions on access to essential medicines.

There is growing appreciation in China for the role of NGOs in many development areas, including AIDS, despite strict controls on civil society registration and activism on politically sensitive matters and limits to institutionalization and scaling up of programmes and services by non-state actors. Moral attitudes stigmatize risk behaviours closely associated with the AIDS epidemic. However transnational NGOs connected to domestic ones have helped carve out a place at the table for AIDS NGOs in China's government-led policy and service provision environment and led to greater acceptance of stigmatized behaviours by society. Local activists connected to global AIDS activism have influenced policies and programmes and helped shape new norms that seemed unheard of only a decade earlier. Such transnational activism is an important mechanism for the globalization of ideas and strategies for advancing social justice and human rights, aided by the internet (Keck and Sikkink 1998, Risse 2000, Florini 2001). In this article, I examine how this process has occurred in China and influenced policy change on several issues.

Background

China's response to its AIDS epidemic during its first two decades was disconnected from global evidence-based policy recommendations and international advice and characterized by nationalism and isolationism. China's first case of AIDS was diagnosed in a South American tourist in 1985 (Yu *et al.* 1996) and subsequently AIDS was labelled as a foreign disease of bad behaviour and immorality not found in China. The illicit behaviours associated with the epidemic by the Chinese public were highly stigmatized – homosexuality, illegal drug use, and prostitution – all considered vices of the West and social problems that had been wiped out by socialist China after 1949 (Cohen *et al.* 1996). The origins of the epidemic (Burmese border) (Beyrer *et al.* 2000) and information about rising infection rates in the 1990s was suppressed by the government, despite urging from international donors, especially UNAIDS, to acknowledge and respond to the epidemic with proven prevention programmes. Official denial characterized this period, while the epidemic was exploding among injecting drug users (IDUs) in China's southwest and reports of a tainted blood donation epidemic in central China were emerging (Rosenthal 2000, Kaufman and Jing 2002). The emerging sexual epidemic among sex workers and homosexual men was downplayed and caught up in official rhetoric of socialist moralism and victim blaming. This period however saw a resurgence of prostitution, rapidly changing sexual behaviours by urban youth, including emergence of an urban community of men who have sex with men (MSM), and a karaoke bar culture for business travellers that extended even to rural market towns (Uretsky 2003, 2008). Evidence about changing attitudes and sexual behaviours among college students (Li *et al.* 1998), abortion among unmarried women (Zhang *et al.* 2000), sexual behaviour surveys, and studies of sex workers (Pan 1999, 2001) during the 1990s did not make their way into AIDS programmes and policies. A few pilot projects reached out to karaoke bars and other sex worker venues with safe sex education and condom promotion, but these pilots were isolated, donor driven and there was no education for the general public through media channels.

Early provincial laws further stigmatized people living with HIV. Chengdu, the capital of populous Sichuan Province in China's southwest, passed a law restricting HIV-infected persons from marrying, serving as kindergarten teachers, surgeons, and other professions, and an early draft proposed prohibiting them from public swimming pools and public baths (Pomfret 2001).

Sex education focused on abstinence promotion for youth (Wan 2000). The promotion of condoms, the only proven method to prevent sexual transmission of HIV at that time, was contested throughout the 1990s, despite advocacy by public health professionals. It was opposed by a public with strongly held Confucian beliefs that sex should not be publicly discussed, especially with girls before marriage. Hard-line moralists in influential positions within the Ministry of Health's Health Education Centre, insisted that condom promotion would lead to promiscuity (Zhou and Chen 2000). A ban on condom advertisements was not lifted until 2003 (Zhang 2002) at which time China reported nearly 1 million people living with HIV in the country.

In 2003, however, China's AIDS policy changed to one of strong national leadership, improved surveillance, and the commitment of substantial domestic resources (US$120 million a year at the national level and US$73 million at the provincial level). An aggressive national prevention and free treatment programme was launched, to deal with the now acknowledged epidemic among rural villagers who donated blood in Central China. Some community-based organizations serving most at risk groups began working with the China Centre for Disease Control (CDC) system to provide services (Wu *et al.* 2007, Zhang *et al.* 2007, Ministry of Health *et al.* 2010). Victim blaming was replaced by aggressive public education campaigns focused on reducing stigma and promoting compassion for people living with HIV and AIDS (PLWHA). Civil society groups, especially those representing MSM and PLWHA gained legitimacy and a place at the table for governance of key donor programmes like the Global Fund to Fight AIDS, TB and Malaria. Criminalization and arrest for IDUs eased with the introduction of a nation-wide harm reduction campaign for IDUs focused on needle and syringe exchange and methadone maintenance therapy. A State Council-led coordination agency, the State Council AIDS Working Committee promotes multi-sectoral coordination and issues policy documents based on global norms (State Council of the People's Republic of China, 2006, 2007, 2010). However, the adoption of some other international norms has been slower to change.

Global governance innovations in the AIDS response

Sidibé *et al.* (2010) have highlighted the significant innovations in global governance for health accompanying the global response to the AIDS epidemic over the last 30 years. These innovations have included: the mobilization of political commitment and accountability for a health issue, including a United Nations General Assembly special session (UNGASS) devoted to the topic; expanded political space for affected persons to participate in governance (the Greater Involvement of Persons Living with HIV and AIDS (GIPA) principle) and planning of the AIDS response (Global Fund CCM, the UNGASS civil society reporting mechanism, UNAIDS 2009a); the use of a human rights discourse to highlight attention to enabling environment requirements (the need to address stigma and discrimination, access to essential medicines); novel institutional mechanisms in the global health architecture (creation of a Global Fund) and innovative new funding mechanisms like UNITAID to guarantee a steady supply of affordable drugs. Global norms and best practices and international agreements have been published and promoted (GIPA Principle, UNAIDS Policy Brief 2007, Paris Declaration 1994) (recent statement on how criminalization interferes with harm reduction approaches to HIV, Vienna Declaration 2010). NGOs and donors have highlighted the critical role that NGOs have played in reaching their constituencies with peer-led AIDS prevention programmes, in providing AIDS treatment adherence support, community-based care, and support for orphans and AIDS-affected communities. International agencies have promoted to governments the importance of creating an enabling environment for effective AIDS programmes, such as anti-discrimination policies. TNCS organizations have at the same time advocated for these best practices and formed alliances with domestic civil society organizations to also push for changes with governments.

A number of mechanisms have helped coalesce the donors, government, and non-government actors around these global norms and build consensus for promoting them as standard practice in national AIDS programmes. The United Nations system and UNAIDS, the joint UN programme that coordinates the work of the UN agencies on AIDS plays a major role. A special UN general assembly session devoted to the AIDS epidemic (UNGASS) has taken place every five years since 2001 and issued a declaration setting out global targets and guidelines (United Nations General Assembly 2001, 2006, 2011). The biyearly International AIDS Conferences and the regional AIDS meetings provide networking opportunities for NGOs working on specific issues and an opportunity for sharing best practices, strategies, and advocacy messages. The rise of the internet has facilitated the ability to maintain virtual networks of these groups and has become a crucial mechanism for the sharing of information both within and between countries and continents.

Global AIDS NGOs, many based in the global south, have played a crucial role in promoting these values and norms around the world. For example, the *Treatment Action Campaign*, a South Africa-based advocacy organization, has played a leading role in advocating for access to essential AIDS medicines, challenging global pharmaceutical companies, through lawsuits and advocacy to bring down the price of AIDS drugs and make them accessible to those who need them in low- and middle-income countries (LMIC). *The Global Network of People Living with HIV and AIDS* (GNP+) has advocated for rights and dignity protection and the enforcement of the GIPA principle globally and at the country level. The Global Business Coalition on AIDS has engaged multinational corporations in corporate social responsibility and workplace programmes based on international standards of confidentiality, non-discrimination, and worker education, collaborated with the International Labour Organization to launch a 'Code of Practice on HIV/AIDS and the world of work' (International Labour Office 2001) and inspired some companies to launch global charitable donation campaigns through product branding and point-of-purchase approaches (e.g. 'Product Red'). At the regional level, networks and alliances of national NGOs have coalesced around such issues as sex worker rights and treatment access. The Global Fund to Fight AIDS, TB and Malaria requires governance by a 'CCM' made up of key national stakeholders including NGOs representing risk groups for the three diseases. The 'call for proposals' on specific topics (e.g. supporting the work of NGOs serving most at risk groups for HIV) and the rules and guidelines of the Fund, are important mechanisms for introducing global priorities and approaches, such as rigorous fiscal management and accountability for fund use.

Transnational connections and civil society organizing on AIDS in China

In the last 20 years China has undergone a major economic and social transformation and is now the world's fastest growing economy. The 'Open Door Policy', adopted by China's political leaders in 1976 has been accompanied by a breakdown in the stringent controls over people's daily lives in the preceding 30 years of austere socialism. China has become an active member in the United Nations and isolationism has given way to an increasing role as global citizen and at times, spokesperson for the developing world. The rise of an economic middle class, especially in more affluent coastal regions, has created greater demand for the protection of individual rights and consumer protection and an evolving rule of law and independent legal system have begun to enforce such rights (even while more constrained in the last few years) more so in urban than rural areas. However, many areas remain off limits for legal recourse, especially sensitive political matters. The growth of the internet, especially blogs (*weibos*) in China has created a relatively open media mechanism for the popularization of ideas and discontents and the rapid spread of information, opinions, and increasingly social action (Yang 2003).

The emergence and growth of civil society is one aspect of movement towards more citizen participation and accountable governance (Saich 2000, 2001, Lee and Hsing 2010), even though its role is highly circumscribed by government (Beja 2008). Despite periodic moves to curtail and restrict civil society organizations, there has been growth and appreciation for their role in many development areas such as the environment, the AIDS response, migrant issues. However strict controls remain on the registration and governance requirements for NGOs (China Development Brief 1998, 1999) and their ability to network and operate beyond narrow locales and/or issue areas or to provide services. Most NGOs remain advocacy or research groups. Financial and political sponsorship are necessary and the required registration is often difficult (Kaufman 2009).

China's civil society sector has grown in a context in which social stability is a dominant theme (Beja 2008) allowing non-combative engagement on a number of issues with the encouragement of the party/state. The political space for engagement is designed and structured by the state, not the groups themselves. Wilson (forthcoming a) invokes Frolic (1997) in describing the China situation as one of 'state-led civil society' and an arena in which state–society relations are negotiated, and where private actors contend with state agents over power and ideas. Examples include how environmental NGOs have prevented dam building in Yunnan Province, how China Global Fund Watch has advocated for greater direct NGO funding for China's AIDS response, or Aizhixing's advocacy for compensation for AIDS victims of Henan Province's unhygienic paid blood donation scheme (see below). These illustrate how civil society groups have been successful in raising attention to important citizens' rights issues through formal dialogue with government organs in a non-confrontational manner. The state allows input into the design of public policies to some degree, speaking the language of governance and engagement of the 'third sector', but full free expression and public debate is circumscribed and the actual governance functions are restricted compared to the power and influence of civil society groups elsewhere.

Connections with and advice from TNCS organizations on a number of sensitive aspects of China's AIDS response has sometimes jump-started or augmented the dialogue between government and domestic NGOs. TNCS groups, working with domestic partners have joined together with national organizations or events to promote global values and approaches influencing local discourse, debate, and in some cases policy change. Internet list serves, chat groups, blogs, and web-based organizing have played an important role. Global list serves like Asia Catalyst and other human rights organizations, regional list serves like SEA-AIDS, and national list serves like China's AIDS NGO-Action have all contributed to a constant stream of information about AIDS activism, events, and hot topics and provided important opportunities for networking and organizing. The greater acceptance of MSM behaviour in China is in large part due to advocacy and activism for AIDS prevention that provided an opening for the hidden and stigmatized MSM community to organize with regional support from MSM groups in Hong Kong and other Asian countries with protection from key academics and intellectuals in China (Zhang and Kaufman 2005, Kaufman 2010, Hildebrant forthcoming).

This 'soft power' approach to global governance has influenced national AIDS policy formulation in China, as it has done elsewhere in the world on other issues (Florini and Simmons 2000). Moreover, even while the political space for NGOs is closely controlled by the state, Chinese government agencies often rely on the expertise of transnationally connected NGOs to advise them on how best to revise their own policies, such as on intellectual property rights and access to essential medicines (discussed below).

Keck and Sikkink (1998) describe how transnational civil society organizing and advocacy (aided by the internet) has led to the globalization of ideas and strategies for advancing aspects of social justice, and Frolic (1997) describes how such processes are operationalized in China through negotiation between state and non-state actors. New ideas and strategies on the AIDS response have been introduced in China through specific mandates for NGO inclusion in governance bodies (e.g. Global Fund), and the transfer of global norms through partnerships of Chinese NGOs with regional or global NGOs, through international conferences, agreements, and multinational organizations working on specific issues. Dialogue with government agencies by domestic NGOs allied with global NGOs, have connected up with donor-led processes to lead to shifts in Chinese government attitudes, policies, and practices on sensitive issues. As noted by Florini and Simmons (2000) TNCS organizing brings with it a moral authority and legitimacy of messages about social justice which provides a 'soft power' to transnational movements. Global norms about the treatment of people living with and affected by HIV and the inclusion of affected and marginalized persons in the response has influenced Chinese policy and has begun to change public attitudes related to AIDS.

I examine a number of issues to illustrate shifts in Chinese social justice attitudes and policy evolution on AIDS, noting in each case limits to wholesale adoption related to China's own cultural norms and attitudes deriving from Confucian belief systems or the tenets of Chinese political culture. These examples illustrate the different ways that TNCS has interacted with domestic civil society, the resulting advocacy to government to promote the adoption of global human rights norms (often in tandem with top-down advocacy by donors or the UN system), progressive government ownership of those norms and values, then reliance on domestic civil society groups for expert technical advice for revising or instituting policy change, and in some cases, inclusion of those same civil society actors in governance and dialogue mechanisms to ensure accountability.

Examples of policy advising and change resulting from transnational civil society organizing

Sex worker representation, organization, and rights protection

China's AIDS response has been relatively weak in the adoption of international norms and approaches for HIV prevention among sex workers (UNAIDS 2009b), but pragmatic discussions that include better protection of sex worker rights has now begun, partly as a result of TNCS organizing supporting the same messages being delivered by UN agencies to the Chinese government. Sex work is widespread in China; even in small cities and towns there are entertainment venues where sexual services can be bought. Most Chinese sex workers are economic migrants seeking work in the booming cities, moonlighting as sex workers or leaving low paying factory jobs for the more profitable sexual services sector, and sending remittances home. Prostitution is a criminal offence in China and highly stigmatized. Public attitudes are influenced by both Confucian moral values about family, women's chastity and proper conduct, and six decades of propaganda about socialist morality. Periodic 'Strike Hard' campaigns are mounted by the police, often prior to major holidays or political events, with popular support. In 2006, the 'Shenzhen Shame Parade' publicly named 100 sex workers whose names, birthdates, and city of origin were publicized before they were sent to re-education centres. A 'Strike Hard' campaign in Beijing on 11 April 2010 involved raiding bars, nightclubs, saunas, and high-end karaoke clubs by more than 8000 police the closing of 256 brothels and detention of 1132 sex workers (Davis and Clarkson 2010). There are 340 detention centres for sex workers around the country (Tucker and Ren 2008, Tucker et al. 2010, ZiTeng 2008).

The 'Asia-Pacific Consultation on HIV and Sex Work', convened by UNAIDS, UNFPA, and the Asia Pacific Network of Sex Workers (APNSW et al. 2010) brought together advocacy organizations (including Chinese NGOs like Ziteng) and HIV policy-makers (including Chinese health officials) to promote rights-based HIV prevention for sex workers. There has been progress on harm reduction for injection drug users in China, also illegal, through the government-sponsored methadone programme (Yin *et al.* 2010), but little similar expansion for sex worker HIV prevention in China, especially through NGOs. Of the 337 NGOs surveyed by China's HIV/AIDS Information Network in 2009, only 9% were focused on sex workers and 7% on drug users, compared to 36% for MSM and 27% for PLWHA (Hui *et al.* 2010). In recent years, through internet networking and support of a US-based NGO, Asia Catalyst, a coalition of groups promoting sex worker rights has come together in China and linked up with the Asia-Pacific Network of Sex Workers and the Global Network of Sex Work Projects to advocate for legal protections and harm reduction programmes for Chinese sex workers. This Chinese Sex Workers' Network involves 12 Chinese organizations and has held two national training workshops for sex worker NGOs in China with technical assistance from its TNCS partners. The China Network organized a protest march in Wuhan (3 August 2010) calling for legalizing sex work and marking 3 August as 'Sex Workers Day', carrying red umbrellas, a symbol employed by the Global Network at the International AIDS Conference in Vienna (Branigan 2010). This recent networking, training, and advocacy to government by sex worker organizations in China, occurring simultaneously with the UN system's promotion of the same norms and principles to the Chinese government about sex worker rights has led China's National AIDS Control Programme (NCAIDS) to focus greater attention on sex workers, especially lower paid workers (Huang 2010) and to explore prevention approaches that have been successful in other Asian countries (Kaufman 2011). Discussion on how to improve policies and programmes for HIV prevention among sex workers has begun.

Inclusion of civil society and participation in governance of the AIDS

The controversy in 2006 surrounding the election of an NGO representative to China's CCM for the Global Fund to fight AIDS, TB and Malaria provided a unique opportunity for advancing international norms about participation of NGOs in the governance of country AIDS responses. The recent suspension of Global Fund moneys to China because of alleged financial irregularities and too limited NGO implementation has also held China accountable to these norms (LaFraniere 2011). The Global Fund programme provided an opening for transnational NGOs to engage with Chinese AIDS NGOs on fair elections – one of the most sensitive political issues in China. The Global Fund was established in 2002 with a mandated governance mechanism requiring establishment of a 'CCM' with civil society representatives (Global Fund 2007), to review, approve, and submit applications. China obtained six rounds of Global Fund funding for AIDS since 2003. While China did establish a CCM, it worked more as a rubber stamp for applications developed and executed by China's Ministry of Health and CDC. Domestic AIDS NGOs had limited voice in the process. The first NGO election in China in 2006 to elect an NGO representative to the CCM was disputed and precipitated a thorough review by the Global Fund and UNAIDS, resulting in a new election that was uniquely transparent, participatory, and accountable (Global Fund Observer 2007). The election, facilitated by the International Republican Institute (IRI), a US NGO that has worked around the world to promote democratic elections, provided an opportunity for internet discussions and networked disparate groups around the country. Several widely attended local meetings brought groups together often for the first time, with IRI, UNAIDS, and donor representatives to teach them how to conduct the elections. The election resulted in two elected representatives and two NGO committees, each constituted with 11 elected representatives from groups representing haemophiliacs, MSM, former plasma donors, and migrant workers (Zhang 2010).

The Global Fund election controversy and resolution served as a door opener for NGO participation in the AIDS response in China, helped to bring on board central government leaders who now (at times grudgingly) accept Global Fund requirements, and established a mechanism, albeit still limited, for voice and input by NGOs into China's AIDS response. Global Fund Round 6 to support HIV prevention by NGOs was seen by many as a further mechanism to institutionalize AIDS NGOs roles in China's AIDS response because all the Fund's contributions were to be dispersed by NGOs rather than government. However its intended implementing agency (principal recipient) was switched at the last moment from a national NGO (China Association for STD and AIDS Prevention and Control) to the government AIDS agency (National Centre for AIDS Prevention and Control of the China CDC). Conditions tied to lifting the suspension of Global Fund moneys included the creation of a new sub-recipient that really represents NGOs (Wong 2011) and a commitment to channel 25% of funding to NGO groups, however whether these reforms will advance are in question now that the Fund's Round 11 has been cancelled. China's recently announced that it would use domestic resources to substitute for cancelled Global Fund moneys and has accelerated a process to contract directly with local NGOs for programme implementation, indicating the government's 'ownership' of this global norm. The acknowledgement of the need for NGO implementation almost certainly has resulted from the initial pressure and requirement from the Fund, the networking and advocacy by the groups themselves aided by external partners like IRI, the HIV/AIDS Alliance, International Council of AIDS Service Organizations, Pact (which has done capacity building), and other international NGOs.

A new NGO, China Global Fund Watch, is monitoring compliance with Global Fund rules and publishes a regular online newsletter, modelled on a similar global organization (AIDSPAN, which publishes the 'Global Fund Observer' online newsletter). China Global Fund Watch played a leading role in publicizing the suspension of AIDS funding to China by the Global Fund and in representing the position of China's grassroots NGOs in calls for reform of the governance mechanism of the China Global Fund grants (Jia 2011, Wong 2011).

Legal protection from employment and educational discrimination

China's cultural context places group rights over individual rights and efforts to protect the rights of individuals with infectious diseases are rarely enforced at local levels if there is a perceived public health benefit associated with restrictions. Such has been the case with both HIV and hepatitis B. Labour practices have included pre-employment screening for hepatitis B and the denial of employment to those who test positive. Students living with HIV have been denied college admission, pregnant women living with HIV have been denied access to hospitals and had their status publicly disclosed. People living with HIV have routinely been denied jobs and in many cases children of HIV positive parents ostracized from primary schools.

Legal and policy prohibitions against employment and educational discrimination is enshrined in international human rights laws including the United Nations Treaty on Economic, Social and Cultural Rights, ratified by the Chinese government in 2001. Global norms applying anti-discrimination statutes to people living with HIV have been promoted through such mechanisms as UNAIDS policy documents on HIV and Human Rights and the International Labour Organization's Code of Practice on HIV/AIDS and the World of Work. China's State Council decrees (2006, 2010) and national AIDS plans (2005, 2011) also include anti-discrimination language. However those rights are rarely enforced through legal mechanisms.

As international human rights law has evolved, transnational human rights groups have increasingly invoked the moral authority of such laws to lobby repressive regimes for reforms (Risse 2000). NGO Groups such as Yirenping, Aizhixing, China Cares, and the China GNP+ alliance have all borrowed strategies from global civil society organizations working on human rights, legal protection from discrimination to advance similar agendas in China, often with funding and technical support of foreign donors and international NGOs. They have been able to gain traction on these issues even in the face of societal stigma towards hepatitis

B and people living with HIV and have pushed for greater legal protections for people living with HIV in both work and school and helped organize legal challenges for specific individuals.

With support from international organizations (and local support from the United Nations Development Programme, UNDP), an alliance of NGO organizations and a public interest law group (Peking University Law School Research Centre for Human Rights and Humanitarian Law 2011) spearheaded a report on 'Anti-Discrimination against HIV/AIDS and Pathogen Hepatitis B Carriers/patients' which examined China's policies and practices in light of international laws, norms, and practices. The alliance identified shortcomings in definitions, enforceability of laws, and pointed out specific regulations, such as the '2008 Guidelines on Physical Check for College Entrance' that discriminate against hepatitis B carriers. Their report provided specific examples from throughout China highlighting cases of discrimination related to the regulations. This influential report led China's Premier Wen Jiabao to call for the amendment of laws and regulations that discriminate against people living with HIV and has resulted in a desk review of Chinese laws and regulations to identify needed changes. The advisory group for the project and ongoing review includes lawyers and leaders of HIV and hepatitis B NGOs (Aizhixing and Yirenping), two groups closely connected to translational human rights networks and transnational NGOs working to enforce legal protections against HIV discrimination in other countries (such as South Africa).

Compensation for accidental HIV infections due to contaminated blood supply

There has been government resistance to acknowledging the legal right to compensation for people living with HIV who acquired the virus through medical negligence, even cancelling an international conference aimed at promoting legal approaches to doing so (Schearf 2007). Yet even this issue has begun to budge. Resistance stems from government's reluctance to opening the door to law suits against government-run health facilities that worked with private blood collectors in central China during the 1990s when many villagers were infected through unclean collection practices. Central Chinese government officials have never admitted responsibility or been held accountable for the hundreds of thousands of inadvertent infections that occurred. Fear of instability and protests have dominated over the moral legitimacy of international norms and the settlements by other governments (e.g. France). In China 'infectious disease sufferers' (i.e. AIDS patients) are even listed by China's public security agency as a category of citizens who might petition higher levels of government and therefore should be monitored by the police to protect social stability (Wan 2011). Even as the courts have resisted and local public security bureaus have strengthened mechanisms to avoid protests and petitions for compensation, some well-connected senior officials including at China's Central Party School, have advocated for compensation for AIDS patients and spearheaded successful court cases.

Several of China's AIDS NGOs with strong connections to transnational human rights networks and transnational NGOs, such as Aizhixing Legal AID Centre, Korekata AIDS Law Centre, Shanghai's Leyi, and some of China's activist public interest lawyers, have tried over many years to represent AIDS patients in the courts to sue for compensation for accidental infections (Wilson forthcoming b). Many of these Chinese groups have participated in legal trainings outside the country and in online forums about international laws and strategies employed in other countries. A leading South African activist and NGO worked with at least one of the groups to provide training and advice. The confluence of global norms, promoted from above and below (the boomerang effect described by Keck and Sikkink 1998), have finally begun to yield movement at the policy level in China. Instigated by UNAIDS, advised by the same South African activist, and organized by one of China's government affiliated NGOs, a 'Red Ribbon Forum' was launched in Beijing in 2010 to create an official dialogue on HIV and human rights between China's AIDS NGO community working on these issues (allied with global human rights networks) and the Chinese government. Funding support comes from China's State Council AIDS Working Committee and UNAIDS and Forum committee members include government law, public security, and health officials, official government led and organized NGOs (GONGOs) working on AIDS and real grassroots AIDS NGOs as well as the activist lawyers themselves. At the third forum meeting in December 2011, the main topic of discussion was the issue of compensation mechanisms for people infected through blood transfusions. One of China's leading human rights lawyers working on HIV and AIDS was invited to draft a compensation plan and is currently assisting in the drafting of a bill to be considered at the Spring 2012 meeting of the Chinese People's Political Consultative Congress – one of the three key law-making bodies in China.

Access to essential medicines and intellectual property rights for essential medicines
A third example illustrates how domestic NGOs linked to transnational groups are working as experts to government to help improve China's policy positions with global institutions on patent rights and intellectual property related to AIDS drugs for its free AIDS treatment programme. The actions of global transnational advocacy networks such as the *Treatment Action Campaign*, a South Africa-based advocacy organization, has played a leading role in advocating for access to essential AIDS medicines, challenging global pharmaceutical companies, through lawsuits and advocacy, and international donors to bring down the price of AIDS drugs and make them accessible to those who need them in LMIC. Such advocacy influenced the World Trade Organization's trade-related aspects of intellectual property (TRIPS) agreement and resulted in the Doha Declaration that excluded drugs needed for public health emergencies from patent protections and allowed countries to use parallel importation or compulsory licensing to meet their needs in such cases. Few countries have taken advantage of these TRIPS flexibilities for fear of trade retaliations. China launched a free national AIDS treatment programme in 2003, relying initially on domestically manufactured off-patent, older, anti-retroviral medicines, and later, acquiring patented medications through direct price negotiations with international pharmaceutical companies or through bulk buying negotiated through groups like the Clinton Foundation.

In recent years, a group of advocates in China have formed an NGO connected to global and regional advocacy groups (the *Third World Network* based in Malaysia and Geneva) working on access to essential medicines. The *China Access to Medicines Research Group* describes itself as a loose civic research network formed by public interest lawyers and public health experts (China Global Fund Watch 2011). They posit that China's reluctance to manufacture patented drugs needed for its treatment programme has resulted in unacceptable levels of low adherence and drug resistance and that the cessation of Global Fund for AIDS, TB, and malaria contributions necessitate urgent action to ensure continued access to AIDS drugs in China. The group has written an open letter to the Ministry of Health, the State Council AIDS Working Committee, and the State Intellectual Property Office (SIPO) calling for sustainable access to AIDS medicines in China and providing specific draft revisions to existing laws on measures for compulsory licensing of patents, comparing original text in the existing regulations to suggested revisions that would ensure greater protection of Chinese citizen's interests (Hu 2011, TWN 2011). These specific blueprints for change are being reviewed by SIPO, and while no official policy change has yet occurred, will likely to be the basis for change when it does occur. This example of how a Chinese civil society group linked to global advocacy networks is providing expert advice to government agencies shows how such groups are assisting in the transfer of global human rights norms for people living with HIV and AIDS.

Conclusion

China's AIDS response has moved from denial and victim blaming to one based more on norms of social justice and inclusion promoted by global policy institutions, even while in some cases at odds with political and cultural attitudes. This change has come about at least in part by a decade or more of TNCS organizing on key sensitive aspects of the AIDS response, greatly facilitated by the expansion of the internet. However, in China's highly constrained political environment, the transfer of global norms and NGO participation in policy formulation and governance occurs in a non-combative way. Because of China's top-down political process and the dominant role of government in policy formulation and service provision, domestic NGOs working with TNCS actors join a bottom-up process to a top-down process through United Nations and other donors to build support for the adoption of global norms and approaches. Beja (2008) noted that political realities have a major influence on how far social movements can progress: the presence and strength of national civil society relative to government will limit achievement of efforts that may be in conflict with national policies.

The expansion of civil society groups in China has progressed in a context in which social stability is a dominant theme, allowing non-combative engagement on a number of issues with the encouragement of the party/state but that political space is designed and structured by the state, not the groups themselves. The state allows input into the design of public policies to some degree, speaking the language of governance and engagement of the 'third sector', but free expression and public debate is circumscribed and the actual governance functions are restricted compared to the power and influence of civil society groups elsewhere. China remains a one-party state with strict controls on civil society activism and strong moral conservatism. However even in such a constrained political and social environment, local activists connected to global AIDS activism and other international actors have influenced policies and programmes and advanced an agenda for rights protection and participation of affected groups.

References

Asia Pacific Network of Sex Workers (APNSW), United Nations Population Fund (UNFPA), and UNAIDS, October 2010. *Asia and the Pacific Regional Consultation on HIV and sex work. Building partnerships on HIV and sex work*. Available from: http://asiapacific.unfpa.org/webdav/site/asiapacific/shared/Publications/2011/Building%20Partnerships%20on%20HIV%20and%20Sex%20Work%202.pdf [accessed 10 April 2012].

Beja, J.-P., 2008. The changing aspects of civil society in China. *In*: Y. Zheng and J. Fewsmith, eds. *China's opening society*. London and New York: Routledge, 71–88.

Beyrer, C., *et al.*, 2000. Overland heroin trafficking routes and HIV-1 spread in South and South-East Asia. *AIDS*, 14 (1), 75–83.

Branigan, T., 2010. Chinese sex workers protest against crackdown. *Guardian*. Available from: http://www.guardian.co.uk/world/2010/aug/03/china-prostitution-sex-workers-protest [accessed 2 October 2011].

China Development Brief, 1998. *Provisional regulations for registration and management of private nonenterprise units*. English-language version. Available from: http://www.chinadevelopmentbrief.com/node/300 [accessed 20 May 2011].

China Development Brief, 1999. *Regulations for registration and management of social organisations*. English-language version. Available from: http://www.chinadevelopmentbrief.com/node/298 [accessed 20 May 2011].

China Global Fund Watch, 2011. Recommendations on sustainable access to HIV medicines in China by Hu Yuanqiang from China Access to Medicines Research Group. Newsletter, Issue No. 17, November 2011, 2–5. China Global Fund Watch Initiative (J. Ping, ed.).

Cohen, M.S., *et al.*, 1996. Successful eradication of sexually transmitted diseases in the People's Republic of China: implications for the 21st century. *Journal of Infectious Diseases*, 174 (Suppl. 2), S223–S229.

Davis, M. and Clarkson, J., 2010. *Beijing launches sweeping crackdown on sex industry*. 26 May. Available from: http://asiacatalyst.org/blog/2010/05/beijing-launches-sweeping-crackdown-on-sex-industry.html [accessed 6 October 2011].

Florini, A.M., 2001. Transnational civil society. *In*: M. Edwards and J. Gaventa, eds. *Global citizen action*. Boulder, CO: Lynne Rienner Publishers Inc, 29–42.

Florini, A.M. and Simmons, P.J., 2000. What the world needs now? *In*: M. Florini, ed. *The third force: the rise of transnational civil society*. Washington, DC: The Brookings Institution Press, 1–15.

Frolic, B.M., 1997. State-led civil society. *In*: T. Brook and B.M. Frolic, eds. *Civil society in China*. Armonk, NY: East Gate Books, 46–47.

Global Fund, 2007. *The global fund overview for East Asia and the Pacific: successes, challenges, and achievements to date*. Geneva: The Global Fund to Fight AIDS, Tuberculosis, and Malaria.

Global Fund Observer, October 2007. *China changes course on using NGOs as grant implementers*. Available from: http://www.aidspan.org/index.php?page=gfo [accessed 5 October 2011].

Hildebrant, T., forthcoming. Development and division: the effect of transnational linkages & local politics on LGBT activism in China. *Journal of Contemporary China*, 21 (76).

Hu, Y., 2011. Recommendations on sustainable access to HIV/AIDS medicines in China. *China Global Fund Watch* Newsletter, Issue No. 17, November 2011. China Global Fund Watch Initiative.

Huang, Y., 2010. Female sex workers in China. *In*: J. Jing and H. Worth, eds. *HIV in China: understanding the social aspects of the epidemic*. Sydney: University of New South Wales Press, 43–65.

Hui, L., et al., 2010. From spectators to implementers: civil society organisations involved in AIDS programmes in China. *International Journal of Epidemiology*, 39 (Suppl. 2), ii65–ii71.

International Labour Office, 2001. *An ILO code of practice on HIV/AIDS and the world of work*. Geneva: International Labour Organisation. Available from: http://www.ilo.org/wcmsp5/groups/public/@ed_protect/@protrav/@ilo_aids/documents/publication/wcms_113783.pdf [accessed 10 April 2012].

Jia, P., 2011. The Global Fund suspended grant disbursement to China Global Fund RCC AIDS program. *China Global Fund Watch Initiative*, 14 (March), 2–5.

Kaufman, J., 2009. The role of NGOs in China's AIDS response – update, challenges and psossibilities. *In*: J. Schwartz and S. Shieh, eds. *Serving the people: State-society negotiations and welfare provision in China*. New York: Routledge, 156–173.

Kaufman, J., 2010. Turning points in China's AIDS response. *China: An International Journal*, 8 (1), 63–84.

Kaufman, J., 2011. HIV, sex work and civil society in China. *Journal of Infectious Diseases*, 204 (Suppl 5), S1218–S1222.

Kaufman, J.A. and Jing, J., 2002. China and AIDS: the time to act is now. *Science*, 296 (5577), 2339–2340.

Keck, M.E. and Sikkink, K., 1998. *Activists beyond borders: advocacy networks in international politics*. Ithaca and London: Cornell University Press.

LaFraniere, S., 2011. AIDS funds frozen for China in grant dispute. *New York Times*, 20 May, p. A4.

Lee, C.K. and Hsing, Y.-T., 2010. Social activism in China: agency and possibility. *In*: Y.-T. Hsing and C.K. Lee, eds. *Reclaiming Chinese society: the new social activism*. London and New York: Routledge, 1–14.

Li, A., et al., 1998. Sexual behaviour and its related psychosocial factors among unmarried university students in Beijing, China. Unpublished report of thesis research for Health and Social Sciences Masters Program, Mahidol University, Thailand.

Ministry of Health of China, Joint United Nations Programme on HIV/AIDS, and World Heath Organization, 2010. *2009 Estimates for the HIV/AIDS epidemic in China*. Available from: http://www.unaids.org.cn/en/index/Document_view.asp?id=413 [accessed 4 October 2011].

Pan, S., 1999. *Three red light districts in China (Zhongguo Guodi Xiaxing Chanye Kaoke)*. Beijing: Qunyan Publishing House.

Pan, S., 2001. AIDS in China: how much possibility is there in sexual transmitting? Unpublished paper. *First China Conference on AIDS/STDs*, Beijing, November 2001.

Peking University Law School, Research Centre for Human Rights and Humanitarian Law, 2011. *Anti-discrimination against HIV/AIDS and pathogen hepatitis B carriers/patients*. Unpublished report, July 2011.

Pomfret, J., 2001. Chinese city's strong measures on HIV and AIDS provoke outcry. *Washington Post*, 16 January. Available from: http://www.iht.com/articles/7601.html [accessed 10 April 2012].

Risse, T., 2000. The power of norms versus the norms of power: transnational civil society and human rights. *In*: A.M. Florini, ed. *The third force: the rise of transnational civil society*. Washington, DC: The Brookings Institution Press, 177–209.

Rosenthal, E., 2000. In rural China, a steep price of poverty: dying of AIDS. *New York Times*, 28 October 2000.
Saich, T., 2000. Negotiating the state: the development of social organisations in China. *The China Quarterly*, 161 (4), 124–141.
Saich, T., 2001. *Governance and politics in China*. Basingstoke: Palgrave.
Schearf, D., 2007. Chinese authorities prevent multinational AIDS Rights Conference. *Voice of America News*, 29 July 2007. Available from: www.asiacatalyst.org/news/inthenews [accessed 10 April 2012].
Sidibé, M., Tanaka, S., and Buse, K., 2010. Innovations in global governance for HIV/AIDS. *Global Health Governance*, IV (1), 1–14.
State Council of the People's Republic of China, 29 January 2006. Regulations on AIDS prevention and control, Decree No. 457.
State Council of the People's Republic of China, 2007. China's action plan for reducing and preventing the spread of HIV/AIDS, 2006–2010, State Council Office Document, No. 13.
State Council of the People's Republic of China, 2010. Notice of the State Council on further strengthening the HIV/AIDS response, Decree (Guo Fa) No. 48.
Third World Network (TWN) and China Access to Essential Medicine Research Group, 2011. Comments on the draft revision of the measures for compulsory licensing on patents. *China Global Fund Watch* Newsletter, Issue No. 17, November 2011. China Global Fund Watch Initiative.
Tucker, J., Ren, X., and Sapio, F., 2010. Incarcerated sex workers and HIV prevention in China: social suffering and social justice countermeasures. *Social Science and Medicine*, 70 (1), 121–129.
Tucker, J.D. and Ren, X., 2008. Sex worker incarceration in the People's Republic of China. *Sexually Transmitted Infections*, 84 (1), 34–35.
UNAIDS, 2009a. *Guidelines on construction of core indicators, 2010 reporting*. Geneva: United Nations General Assembly Special Session on HIV/AIDS (UNGASS).
UNAIDS, 2009b. *UNAIDS global guidance on HIV and sex work*. Available from: http://data.unaids.org/pub/BaseDocument/2009/jc1696_guidance_note_hiv_and_sexwork_en.pdf [accessed 19 May 2011].
UNAIDS Policy Brief, March 2007. *The Greater Involvement of People Living with HIV*. GIPA, UNAIDS - Joint United Nations Programme on HIV/AIDS, Geneva, Switzerland.
United Nations General Assembly, 2001. Declaration of commitment on HIV/AIDS, 2 August 2001, A/Res/S-26-2. Available from: www.un.org/ga/aids/docs/aress262.pdf [accessed 10 April 2012].
United Nations General Assembly, 2006. Political declaration on HIV/AIDS, 15 June 2006, A/Res/60/262. Available from: http://data.unaids.org/pub/report/2006/20060615_hlm_politicaldeclaration_ares60262_en.pdf) [accessed 10 April 2012].
United Nations General Assembly, 2011. Implementation of the declaration of commitment on HIV/AIDS and the political declaration on HIV/AIDS, 8 June 2011, A/65/L77. Available from: www.un.org/ga/search/view_doc.asp?symbol=A/65/L.77 [accessed 10 April 2012].
Uretsky, E., 2003. Research note: the importance of research on male sexuality in China for effective HIV/AIDS prevention programs. *Yale-China Health Journal*, 2 (Autumn), 45–53.
Uretsky, E., 2008. 'Mobile men with money': the socio-cultural and politico-economic context of high-risk behavior among wealthy businessmen and government officials in urban China. *Culture, Health, and Sexuality*, 10 (8), 801–814.
Vienna Declaration, 2010. The criminalisation of illicit drug users is fuelling the HIV epidemic and has resulted in overwhelmingly negative health and social consequences. A full policy reorientation is needed. Available from: http://www.viennadeclaration.com/the-declaration/ [accessed 4 October 2011].
Wan, Y., 2000. *Diedao de muyangren: xingqunjie jiaoyu he xing anchuan jiaoyu bijiao yanjiu, dui guoji jiaoyu jijinghui he tongyi jiaohui de yanjiu* [The fallen shepherd: comparative study of abstinence education and sexual health education and study on the International Education Foundation and the Unification Church]. Bejing, China: AIZHI Action Project.
Wan, Y., 2011. Political stability, health, and rights in China. Unpublished presentation at *Fordham University Law School Conference on AIDS in China*, 24 February 2011.
Wilson, S., forthcoming a. Introduction: Chinese NGOs – international and online linkages. *Journal of Contemporary China*, 21 (76).
Wilson, S., forthcoming b. Seeking one's day in court: Chinese regime responsiveness to international legal norms on AIDS carriers' and pollution victims' rights. *Journal of Contemporary China*, 21 (77).
Wong, G., 2011. AP News Break: Global Fund lifts China grant freeze. *The Associated Press*, 23 August. Available from: www://news.yahoo.com/apnewsbreak-global-fund-lifts-china-grant-freeze-131838094.html [accessed 10 October 2011].

Wu, Z.Y., et al., 2007. Evolution of China's response to HIV/AIDS. *Lancet*, 369, 679–690.
Yang, G., 2003. The co-evolution of the internet and civil society in China. *Asian Survey*, 43 (3), 405–422.
Yin, W., et al., 2010. Scaling up the national methadone maintenance treatment program in China: achievements and challenges. *International Journal of Epidemiology*, 39 (Suppl. 2), ii29–ii37.
Yu, E., et al., 1996. HIV infection and AIDS in China, 1985 through 1994. *American Journal of Public Health*, 86 (8), 1116–1122.
Zhang, B. and Kaufman, J., 2005. The rights of people with same sex sexual behavior: recent progress and continuing challenges in China. *In*: G. Misra and R. Chandiramani, eds. *Sexuality, gender and rights: exploring theory and practice in south and South East Asia*. New Delhi: Sage Publications, 113–130.
Zhang, F., 2002. Ban on condom ads set to go. *China Daily*, 2 December.
Zhang, F., et al., 2007. The Chinese free antiretroviral treatment program: challenges and responses. *AIDS*, 21 (Suppl 8), S143–S148.
Zhang, T., 2010. New paradigm of grassroots participation in governance: Research on the First China Global Fund NGO Work Committee (2007–2009). Unpublished paper 2010.
Zhang, Z., Cao, X., and Zhang, W. (Tianjin Family Planning Institute), 2000. The analysis of sexual knowledge, attitude and behavior among teenagers, *Proceedings of the International Symposium on Reproductive Health Research and Policy Issue of Adolescent and Unmarried Young Adults*, Shanghai Institute for Planned Parenthood Research/WHO, Shanghai China, 19–21 October 2000.
Zhou, Q. and Chen, Y., 2000. Roundtable discussion on sex education for youth. *Greenapple: Adolescent Education Journal*, 4, 7–8.
ZiTeng, 2008. Commentary. *Sexually Transmitted Infections*, 84, 36.

Lessons from the rise and fall of the military AIDS hypothesis: politics, evidence and persuasion

Michael O'Keefe

This article traces the genus of an idea whose time has past, but provides enduring lessons for public policymaking on HIV and AIDS. The focus is on an AIDS myth that quickly became an orthodoxy, but did not stand close scrutiny and was upturned by a lack of evidence. However, its significance in reshaping international public policy has outlived its marginalisation and it stands as a study of a largely political dynamic that if repeated could be counterproductive to ongoing efforts to combat the AIDS epidemic.

Introduction

This article is written in the context of reviews of the legacy of securitisation and sober reappraisals that have prompted a shift away from this perspective (McInnes 2009, McInnes and Rushton 2010, Smith and Whiteside 2010). In particular, it seeks to highlight that the debate may have shifted, but that the implications for marshalling resources are ongoing. This article *does not* seek to enter the wider debate over the securitisation of AIDS that is covered extensively in the literature (see, for instance, Save the Children 2002, Williams 2003, Elbe 2006). Securitisation is a much broader issue of which the military AIDS hypothesis forms one part.

The focus of this article is the significance of the argument that military HIV infection rates were higher than the general public, that through AIDS this had significant national security impacts, and that it in turn it had regional and international security implications. This relationship is termed the 'military AIDS hypothesis' from here on and is treated as an important AIDS myth.

The military AIDS hypothesis was an important part of broader debates because it buttressed parallel arguments that together promoted securitisation. It has been a significant public policy issue because the practical implications of accepting the military AIDS hypothesis were that the international community should target the spread of AIDS in, and by, militaries. The myth became an orthodoxy in the early 2000s and it became institutionalised. However, the important role of the hypothesis in placing HIV and AIDS at the centre of the international security agenda was not simply the resources attracted to prevention among militaries. These were minor in comparison to the rapid scaling up of global efforts to respond to the epidemic. The significance of the military AIDS hypothesis was that the spill over effect of securitisation led to a rapid expansion in resources to broader efforts to combat AIDS and, in an environment where resources are becoming scarce, the fact that the hypothesis was discredited provides lessons for future efforts to attract attention and resources to combating HIV and AIDS.

In order to trace the role of the military AIDS hypothesis in buttressing the broader securitisation of AIDS this article begins with a note on the context behind the shift and then moves to discussion of the political and evidential foundations of the argument. It then reviews the rise of the hypothesis as a justification for prioritising international efforts to combat the epidemic and then concentrates on the cracks that appeared in the foundations and their implications for the securitisation of HIV and AIDS in international public policy.

Context: the rise of the military AIDS hypothesis as a justification for prioritising international efforts to combat the epidemic

The hypothesis that AIDS in militaries had significant security implications coalesced in the late 1990s to early 2000s. It was based on a growing *belief* among some influential policymakers, academics and practitioners in the field. Throughout the 1990s the literature on the impact of HIV and AIDS deepened and broadened (see, for instance, Civil Military Alliance to Combat HIV and AIDS various years, Ogba 1989, Fitzsimons and Whiteside 1992). The dramatic geopolitical changes wrought by the end of the Cold War allowed reappraisals to occur and new perspectives, such as human security, to become more popular (Chen *et al.* 2003, Altman 2008a, 2008b), especially among NGOs (Carballo *et al.* 2002, Centre for Conflict Resolution 2005). This shift should not be overstated. The bulk of the international relations literature remained focused on traditional issues while on the margins there was a proliferation of new transnational or 'soft' security studies that concentrated on issues that had hitherto been absent from mainstream discussion.

The security agenda broadened to include population flows, environmental issues, gender, transnational crime and epidemic diseases. However, HIV and AIDS was but one issue in a crowded agenda and often only rated a brief mention. For example, in *International Relations in the New Century* the chapter on 'Pandemic threats to security' included half a page on war and conflict and half a page on changing human behaviour (read HIV), but the two issues were not directly connected (Chalk 2001, pp. 183–184, Dupont 2001a).

The idea that there were significant links between AIDS and conflict had been coalescing but had not led to concrete action. By 2000 the landscape changed swiftly. The over-arching argument was that causal links existed between AIDS and conflict in sub-Saharan Africa (Mills 2000, Fourie and Schonteich 2001, Ostergard 2002, Heinecken 2003). Initially the discussion was limited to Africa, but the argument became geographically generalised (Hsu 2001, Dupont 2001b, Sokhey 2004).

The causal link between militaries and AIDS was that soldiers (uniformed personnel, peacekeepers, militias and other irregular combatants) were not only at a greater risk of infection than the general public but also that soldiers were significant vectors in the spread of the disease (Conflict, Security & Development Group 2000, Goyer 2001, Tripodi *et al.* 2001, DeWaal 2002, Foreman 2002, Bazergan 2003). This contention was a key element in the securitisation of AIDS and it was repeated in significant articles on the subject.

Through securitisation and international institutionalisation this idea quickly became an orthodoxy. In fact, the securitisation of AIDS was buttressed by the contention that militaries were key vectors in the spread of the virus. It is the implications of this buttressing, especially when it was found to be an illusory foundation, that forms the focus of this paper.

The political birth of securitisation through the military AIDS hypothesis

If a moment in time could capture the change in how HIV and AIDS was perceived by politicians and policymakers it would be the UN Security Council's (UNSC's) Session on AIDS in Africa in January 2000. The USA held the Presidency of the Security Council and Richard Holbrooke, the

Permanent Representative of the USA to the UN, provided leadership that turned the contention that there were close links between AIDS and conflict into an international public policy reality.

Holbrooke is clear that the issue of HIV transmission by, and infection among, peacekeepers in Cambodia in the early 1990s strongly influenced his commitment to elevating the security implications of HIV and AIDS to the forefront of international public policy:

> It is the cruellest of ironies that every time we vote to establish a peacekeeping mission, we are unintentionally helping to spread a killer disease. (UN 2001, p. 11)

Al Gore's speech to the assembled dignitaries at the UNSC Session epitomises the change and its urgency. The Vice President of the most powerful nation on earth epitomised the mood when he made a direct connection between AIDS and national and international security thus broadening the definition of security and the mandate of the UN.

> AIDS is not just a humanitarian crisis. It is a security crisis – because it threatens not just individual citizens but the very institutions that define and defend the character of a society. (2000, p. 1)

Securitising HIV and AIDS in this manner was unprecedented. This was the first time that a 'soft' security issue had crossed into the traditional security concerns of states. Other public health issues (such as Severe Acute Respiratory Syndrome, SARS) have followed, but the ground was broken by the way in which a disease specific response to international security gained emphasis and dedicated funding so quickly.

Gore (2000) was referring to sub-Saharan Africa, but the broader implications were clear. The link to militaries was established by asserting that 'it strikes the military, and subverts the forces of order and peacekeeping' (p. 2). UN Secretary General Kofi Anan and others present also highlighted the connections between HIV in uniformed forces and security threats (Anan 2000). Furthermore, Gore connected the issue to the 'largest-ever increase in' USA spending on AIDS programmes. Another major new announcement was that the US military would cooperate with foreign militaries to combat the epidemic in their ranks. This was a new 'combat' role for the US military and one that added another dimension to the securitisation of the issue. It was followed by a range of initiatives, most notably George Bush Administration's President's Emergency Plan for AIDS Relief (PEPFAR), which allowed billions of dollars to be directed to priority areas for the Administration of the day (Dietrich 2007).

Having the US Vice President (and future Presidential hopeful) mount a case at a special session of the UNSC legitimised the military AIDS hypothesis. Piot, the Executive Director of the Joint United Nations Programme on HIV/AIDS (UNAIDS), noted that: 'The simple fact that the world's ultimate tribunal on questions of peace and security devotes its attention to AIDS sends a very powerful message' (UN 2001, p. 6).

Legitimisation in the UN led to institutionalisation by various high-level intergovernmental meetings focussed on AIDS and security that followed in 2000–2001. These include, but were not limited to, the UNAIDS sponsored strategy meetings between civilian and military experts, the Economic Commission for Africa's African Development Forum on *AIDS: The Greatest Leadership Challenge*, the UN General Assembly Special Session and *Declaration of Commitment on HIV/AIDS*, and *Asia Pacific Ministerial Meeting on HIV/AIDS and Development in Asia and the Pacific*. Furthermore, at this time the issue of AIDS as a security issue was on the agenda or discussed at a range of other important regional meetings, such as the G8 in Okinawa, the Caribbean Community, the Association of Southeast Asian Nations and the Organisation of African Unity. The notion that the epidemic should be treated as a security issue had gained international momentum.

In addition to diplomatic recognition and cooperation, unprecedented interagency cooperation began within the UN (UNAIDS, UN Department of Peacekeeping Operations, UN Economic and Social Commission, UN Development Programme, UN Children's Fund,

UN Population Fund, etc.) and between these agencies and other inter-governmental organisations (such as WHO) and individual states. Tangible outputs of this cooperation occurred quickly, through alterations to UN peacekeeping operations and reports such as the Inter Agency Standing Committee's *Guidelines for HIV/AIDS Interventions in Emergency Settings* (Inter Agency Standing Committee (IASC) 2004). The military AIDS hypothesis became entrenched in international public policymaking.

A dramatic increase in funding occurred from donor countries and organisations, such as the Bill and Melinda Gates Foundation, to ensure that international public heath priorities shifted to target the epidemic, but importantly military issues formed only a small component of this approach. That is, the significance of the military AIDS hypothesis was not that resources flowed into dealing with military prevention but that it helped justify a dramatic increase in resources applied to countering the epidemic.

Broadening the political consensus by bringing African epidemics home (metaphorically at least)

An essential aspect of securitisation through the military AIDS hypothesis was to anchor the argument in the interests of potential detractors on the Security Council and to broaden the consensus by bringing the (potentially) catastrophic impacts of the epidemic to the 'home' constituencies of donors. This helps explain the why the dynamic of state failure and HIV and AIDS in sub-Saharan Africa gained such prominence, and also why the link was made to peacekeepers – as vectors of the disease in host states, but also as victims who would bring the epidemic 'home' to donor states (for instance, for Canada, see Harker 2001, pp. 6–7).

If the implications for African militaries and states were not concrete enough, the peacekeeping aspect of the military AIDS hypothesis had clear implications for non-African states involved in peacekeeping (Barnett and Prins 2006, pp. 367–368). UNSC Resolution 1308 was a key plank in the securitisation of AIDS and the threat to and from peacekeepers was essential to justifying the relevance of the epidemic to the UN mandate. Thus the focus of 1308 was on preparing and protecting peacekeeping personnel through prevention efforts (UN 2000, Bazergan 2004), and this was justified by the military AIDS hypothesis. From then on every peacekeeping resolution referred to the need to train peacekeepers in HIV awareness and these prevention efforts have been highly effective.

From early on in there was debate over whether it was advisable to use peacekeeping as a justification for ramping up HIV prevention efforts. That is, whether the Security Council mandate should deal with health threats (David 2001). Support in the UNSC for broadening its mandate to include health issues was not complete but careful US diplomacy ensured the resolution passed (McInnes and Rushton 2010). The role of Holbrooke in steering resolution 1308 into a central place in the history of AIDS highlights that the birth of the military AIDS hypothesis was essentially political.

We could speculate about the motives of political leaders involved in agenda setting, but a definitive account is almost impossible to construct due to the numbers of actors and competing and contradictory explanations for their behaviour. For the purposes of this article the motives of political leaders count, but do not change the fact that Resolution 1308 was essentially a political response to a health emergency, and one that had unprecedented ramifications for how HIV and AIDS would be perceived, treated and funded. Key US and UN figures provided leadership to ensure that the epidemic took centre stage in international security considerations, which led to a dramatic increase in resources allocated to combating the epidemic. As such, politicians and policymakers set the agenda and others followed. What of the evidence for the military AIDS hypothesis that buttressed the elevation of AIDS as an international security issue?

The evidence supporting the political agenda to securitise AIDS

US diplomatic leadership provided credibility and attention to an issue that had hitherto had low or no profile at the highest levels of international policymaking. AIDS certainly had never been treated as an international security issue before. Proponents of securitisation through the military AIDS hypothesis were able speak authoritatively because they were relying on what they assumed was the credible evidence produced by the US Department of Defense.

In 2000 the US National Intelligence Council (NIC) released the most influential evidence of the links between the epidemic, military forces and conflict. The NIC (2000) report, *The Global Infectious Disease Threat and Its Implications for the United States*, became the mainstay for the securitisation of HIV and AIDS. This report was unprecedented in that it argued that national security and international peacekeeping were threatened by the growing AIDS epidemic. It argued that causal links between the epidemic and military readiness and capability were significant and worthy of attention. It also suggested that links existed between the epidemic and political instability, insecurity and conflict. Furthermore, it noted that peacekeepers were susceptible to infectious disease and were vectors in their spread, the implication being that the capacity of the international community to respond to instability would be diminished by the epidemic.

Militaries were targeted as a key problem:

> Infectious diseases will affect national security and international peacekeeping efforts as militaries and military recruitment pools experience death and disabilities from infectious diseases. The greatest impact will be among hard-to-replace officers, non-commissioned officers, and enlisted soldiers with specialised skills. (2000)

Table 1 was included as evidence to support the preceding claims.

The implications of this table appeared clear and it provided the foundation upon which policymakers would elevate the epidemic to the level of a national security priority (and ultimately an international security priority).

This represented a major shift in the approach by the US security establishment to the epidemic. For instance, a classified Central Intelligence Agency (CIA) report into the implications of AIDS in sub-Saharan Africa from 1987 makes no connection to broader security issues (CIA 1987). This report reflected the thinking at the time, but the NIC report did more than reflect a consensus; it actually led the way in the securitisation of the epidemic through the military AIDS hypothesis. The NIC report's title highlights the focus of the report on US interests '... *Its Implications for the United States*'. The essential fact that the report was born in the US political and security establishment and designed to influence that audience should not be overshadowed by subsequent events where the implications were generalised. To this background the NIC statement had even more significance. Where the US security establishment leads, others often follow and thus the military AIDS hypothesis influenced the militaries of the developed

Table 1. HIV prevalence in selected militaries in sub-Saharan Africa.

Country	Estimated HIV prevalence (%)
Angola	40–60
Congo (Brazzaville)	10–25
Cote d'Ivoire	10–20
Democratic Republic of the Congo	40–60
Eritrea	10
Nigeria	10–20
Tanzania	15–30

Source: DIA/AFMIC (1999).

world and beyond. As such, some of the most conservative governmental institutions were convinced of the seriousness of countering the epidemic.

Another important subsidiary document that led to the 2000 announcement was the May 1998 UNAIDS statement on *AIDS and the Military*. This report epitomised the approach that established the scope of the military AIDS hypothesis. It used circumstantial evidence to buttress the military AIDS hypothesis. This was namely that militaries face a range of risk factors that make them susceptible to HIV infection (age, sex, ethos of risk taking, opportunities for risky behaviour, separation from community and use of sex workers). It also extrapolated the significance of the higher prevalence rates that the risk factors would cause. These were: degrading military capacity and preparedness, increasing infection rates in the broader community, especially in relation to civilian populations at home and when operating abroad (UNAIDS 1998).

Finally, *AIDS and the Military* provided a range of concrete recommendations for action. The provision of recommendations for developing an effective response supported the subsequent institutionalisation of the military AIDS hypothesis. The hypothesis was institutionalised through the international cooperation mentioned above, increased funding and the effective mainstreaming of military prevention efforts (such as prevention education, condom promotion and provision and testing and counselling) (e.g. Healthlink 2002, Sokhey 2004, Lancet 2010).

In the late 1990s and early 2000s the political will was decisive, the evidence appeared strong, the argumentation clear; the military AIDS hypothesis appeared a worthy driver of policy. This was an endearing argument as militaries have been long regarded as susceptible to infectious diseases, in particular sexually transmitted infections and the risk factors in relation to HIV seemed comprehensive and convincing (Hankins *et al.* 2002).

This article now turns to review how the military AIDS hypothesis initially became entrenched in international studies. That is, it traces how the myth escaped its essentially political lineage to become orthodoxy among the academic analysts of the international public policy of HIV and AIDS.

Turning a mirage into an illusion

With Resolution 1308 the connections between AIDS and conflict gained significant attention among political leaders. It is at this point that the (nascent) epidemiological evidence made the 'jump' to international studies literature. This is not to suggest that some academic sources from the late 1990s and 2000s did not mirror the arguments produced by NIC and UNAIDS (Kingma 1996, Yeager *et al.* 2000), but they had not gained political traction or led to the international institutionalisation of a dramatically scaled up response to the epidemic.

Over a short period of time numerous articles appeared establishing the academic credentials of the military AIDS hypothesis. Altman, Eberstadt, Elbe, Singer and other authors mentioned elsewhere in this article reached the same conclusions (Eberstadt 2002, Elbe 2002, Singer 2002, Altman 2003).

Representative examples include Elbe's and Singer's work. They cited the NIC's evidence to paint a bleak picture of the serious international and national security threats posed by the epidemic.

> AIDS not only threatens to heighten the risks of war, but also multiplies its impact. The disease will hollow out military capabilities, as well as state capacities in general, weakening both to the point of failure and collapse ... jeopardising certain pillars of international stability. (Singer 2002, pp. 145–146)

As with most publications during this time Elbe and Singer highlighted the usual factors that formed the military AIDS hypothesis: higher than average prevalence rates ('around four times' the general population); combat effectiveness being degraded; strategic capacity being eroded (both recruits and skilled manpower); peacekeeping operations being complicated; and peacekeeping as a vector in the spread of HIV both at home and abroad (Elbe 2002, Singer 2002).

A review of the literature reveals that the few sources of evidence mentioned above were repeatedly cited to make the case for accepting the military AIDS hypothesis (see previous note and Heinecken 2001, Hsu 2001, Tripodi et al. 2001, Dupont 2001a, 2001b, Schneider and Moodie 2002, Sarin 2003). The source given as the sole justification by most articles was *The Global Infectious Disease Threat and Its Implications for the United States* (NIC 2000). In particular the NIC table of prevalence rates in African militaries above was reproduced numerous times. The academic sources from the late 1990s that mirrored the arguments produced by NIC and UNAIDS were similarly repeatedly cited (Kingma 1996, Yeager et al. 2000).

The consensus in the international studies on the significance of the epidemic meant that academic work became aligned with the politically sponsored institutionalism of AIDS as a security issue. There was a political and academic consensus backed by unprecedented international institutionalisation.

Cracks in the edifice: the rise of 'Securitisation Revisionists'

The military AIDS hypothesis was endearing in that it was supported by early epidemiological studies, anecdotal evidence and academic argument. The problem was that hypotheses need to be tested to be proven, and in this case the essential causal links were not reviewed (or could not be reviewed due to problems with the evidence base). Just because soldiers are placed in very risky situations does not mean that they get infected with HIV at higher rates than the general population. The AIDS epidemic had the potential to be a destabilising force (especially in already fragile states) but had this actually occurred?

Many of the sub-Saharan countries where the epidemic was serious and growing also experienced conflict, but often the evidence was not clear and the narrative was often speculative. That is, a supposed connection between the epidemic and conflict was identified but the causal link between military infection rates and a growing epidemic was not established. That being said, a mix of eclectically produced prevalence rates and estimates and risk factors for soldiers proved a potent force and was repeatedly cited.

As the 2000s wore on more critical perspectives began to be aired. All the key claims that rose to prominence in 2000 were challenged. A representative example of this reappraisal was Whiteside et al.'s (2006) 'AIDS, Security and the Military in Africa: A Sober Reappraisal'. They targeted what they termed the AIDS 'shibboleths' of securitisation. They questioned whether there was higher prevalence among militaries, whether AIDS degraded the functioning of militaries, whether sexual violence during conflict accelerated the spread of the disease, and the strategic question of whether the epidemic had international security implications. They found that most discussion of these issues was speculative assertion based on evidence that may not be generalisable (Whiteside et al. 2006).

The validity of the military AIDS hypothesis as a buttress for the securitisation of AIDS was questioned. For example, Garrett's (2005) influential Council on Foreign Relations report argued that there was a problem with HIV and AIDS in militaries that demanded attention, but that this reflected the epidemic in the general population. In addition, Lowicki-Zucca et al. (2009) sought to refute the peacekeeping aspect and found that prevalence was lower than the populations of host countries.

Work by McInnes (2006), Becker et al. (2008), etc. added to the debate by acknowledging that there was no proven causal link between AIDS and instability. However, like Whiteside et al. above, McInnes did not completely jettison the possible connections, and argued that they were not as simple as initially suggested. So, the debate among those initially supportive of securitisation shifted to the more complex links that they argued still existed. However, how this was to be done was unclear considering the absence of new evidence on the public record of prevalence rates in militaries. Furthermore, it was beginning to become apparent that securitisation may have had unintentional negative consequences; 'an overriding focus on conflict as a vector for HIV not only oversimplifies the epidemiology of the disease but may lead to other major vectors being ignored or not given sufficient attention' (McInnes 2006, p. 325).

Many commentators referred to the lack of evidence or lack of robustness of the original NIC data (Elbe 2003, p. 29, Bazergan 2004, pp. 6–7). The implication was that anecdotal observations and statistical estimates were formed in the absence of accurate and comprehensive epidemiological data. This method of assigning priority to public policy issues was not sustainable in the long term. For instance, Barnett and Prins' influential report to UNAIDS, which was simultaneously published in a leading international relations journal, advocated caution to the background of increased international emphasis on AIDS as a security issue. Barnett and Prins (2006) explicitly acknowledged that, 'asserted statistics about high prevalence in uniformed forces tended to be recycled from one secondary source to another'. The conclusion was that more research needed to be done to identify causal links between HIV, conflict (and uniformed services). Significantly, they also did not reject the link between AIDS and conflict, only the evidence used to make this assertion. More evidence was required but it never materialised on the public record.[1]

It might be useful to give these academics, policymakers and practitioners a label. They could be termed 'securitisation revisionists'. They were clear that most of the causal links that the military AIDS hypothesis was based on were unintentionally misleading; non-existent, weak or unsubstantiated. However the implication was not that the securitisation argument had no merit whatsoever. Most highlighted that while unproven, some connection between AIDS and conflict existed and should still be pursued (Becker *et al.* 2008). Others, such as McInnes (2011), acknowledged 'that HIV prevalence does not always increase in conflict and that in some instances it may even reduce'.

McInnes (2009) moved the debate forward by searching for alternative connections between HIV and AIDS and conflict focusing on susceptibility and vulnerability. The implication was that the military AIDS hypothesis was now so qualified as to make it one of many explanations rather than an over-riding justification for international and national public policy.

As the second decade of the twenty-first century dawned the academic proponents had largely reappraised the initial support for securitisation through the military AIDS hypothesis. The situation was seen to be much more complex and context dependent. The generalisability of 'evidence' was replaced with case specific analyses. The new diffuse orthodoxy was a much more nuanced account of the relationship between AIDS and security.

The military AIDS hypothesis was significant in so for as it had buttressed the securitisation of AIDS and influenced international and national policies countering HIV and AIDS for over a decade despite its weak evidential foundations. It had had appeal because it had strong political support, was institutionalised in the international public heath architecture, was intuitive, and backed by seemingly solid epidemiological evidence and social science argumentation. However, this was not enough to ensure its longevity and by the late 2000s the military AIDS hypothesis had been refuted by academic scrutiny.

The evidence gap and securitisation

The natural implication of the catastrophisation of the impact of AIDS in the early 2000s should have been to undertake more research into military prevalence rates in sub-Saharan Africa.

However, other than a few notable studies, such as Spiegel's work, this sort of sustained seroprevalence work has not been published (Speigel *et al.* 2007). The lack of updated information was a warning of the essentially political basis of the hypothesis. A range of issues will be canvassed below to contextualise the problem.

There were problems with the lack of data and with the scope and quality of the data available. There were many reasons for this, not least that conflict could limit capacity to collect data. Furthermore, this lack of data, etc. mirrored the situation in relation to data on the epidemic more broadly in the early 2000s. However, this does not adequately explain the evidence gap, especially considering the fact that comprehensive, reliable and comparable data on non-military aspects of the epidemic became available over the course of the 2000s.

During the 2000s major prevention efforts occurred in militaries in developed countries (Bing 2005), but these forces were never the focus of the military AIDS hypothesis. Furthermore, the fact that studies did occur highlights the emphasis the developing world places on soldiers from 'home', which reflects the central place of peacekeeping as a justification for securitisation mentioned earlier.

Only a few states conducted annual compulsory testing and again most of these were developed states that are not the focus of this article. Many states conducted pre-employment testing and some conducted pre-deployment testing for peacekeepers (Yeager *et al.* 2000). States also had various approaches to dealing with positive results (Healthlink 2002). For instance, some states used positive HIV status as a reason for precluding entry into the military.

These variations in the approach taken by individual states had a direct impact on the generalisability of data. For instance, peacekeeping was a key justification for the efforts of Holbrooke and others to securitise the epidemic through the Security Council. The lessons from Cambodia and other operations were used to justify action (Elbe 2003, p. 41). However, due to gaps in testing it is not clear whether the infection rates of returning soldiers meant that they contracted HIV there or whether they brought it home. That is, pre-deployment testing was not always undertaken so either inference was not necessarily sustained by the evidence.

Furthermore, some states used HIV positive status as a reason for discontinuing service. This limited the impact of studies that focused on testing of recruits because the results do not necessarily acknowledge that pre-employment testing does not necessarily reflect seroprevalence within militaries (Oumar *et al.* 2008). That is, pre-recruitment testing shows the rate of HIV among the pool of potential recruits and this reflected the rate in that group in the general population; it is not surprising that HIV infection among 18–24-year-old male recruits was higher than the general population. However, sub-Saharan militaries may not have employed HIV positive applicants so rates of infection in militaries could actually have be lower in this age group than in the general population.

Another problem is that *if* data existed for sub-Saharan states it was not generally released on the public record due to its sensitive national security implications (Elbe 2002, p. 165). In the early 2000s, Jean-Marie Guehenno, the Under-Secretary General for Peacekeeping Operations, noted that even when there is post-deployment testing 'National governments do not, as a matter of practice, inform the United Nations that one of their personnel have contracted HIV while on mission' (UN 2001, p. 3. Bazergan 2004, p. 6). In the late 2000s, the US Department of Defense argued that this was because militaries did not publish their prevalence rates or even estimates, but this was not convincing for a number of reasons. Department of Defense publications contradicted this claim. For instance, Department of Defense HIV/AIDS Prevention Programme (DHAAP) (2005) reports regularly noted statements such as: 'Although Zambia has not performed HIV surveillance to determine infection rates amongst ZDF members, infection rates are believed to be 35%, which is significantly higher than the civilian population' (p. 74) This was a dramatic decline from the 1998 estimates of 60% and was listed under the heading 'Winning Battles against HIV/AIDS', but there was no suggestion that there had been a drop from the initial estimates because their credibility was questionable. Furthermore, similar comments were made about numerous countries such as Democratic Republic of the Congo, Nigeria, Swaziland, Tanzania, etc. (DHAAP 2005).

The lack of baseline data meant that longitudinal analysis could not occur. Researchers could not answer the question of whether initial estimates were proven to be correct and/or whether the situation got worse or improved over time. Furthermore, cross-country comparisons could not be made. Therefore researchers did not have the data needed to review the impact of the epidemic on sub-Saharan states.

This evidence gap was described by DeWaal (2002) as a 'huge chasm from which virtually no information has escaped: the military itself' (p. 88). This lack of comprehensive data limited the generalisability of what data were available (van den Assum and Rajbhandari 2005, p. 9).

Not only was there a lack of information in the 2000s, DHAAP reports also catalogued the almost complete lack of military testing and surveillance infrastructure in sub-Saharan Africa before 2001 (DHAAP 2005, 2009). By 2008 even the NIC conceded 'the risks of the disease may have been overstated' (NIC 2008, p. 29). Estimates were produced from very small samples relating to very specific circumstances and populations (that is with limited generalisability). The clear implication was that the figures in the *Global Infectious Disease Threat* widely missed the mark (DHAAP 2005, 2009).

Nowhere was an explanation provided for where the NIC got the estimates it used to brief the US Government. Furthermore, under the heading 'A Word About Data', the original NIC report acknowledged these deficiencies, but rested its conclusions on the assumption that cases were 'unreported or under-reported'. This assumption has proven questionable and the fact that estimates were biased towards exaggerating the threat has been evidenced elsewhere (O'Keefe 2011). In addition, the significance for epidemiologists of this caveat to the original figures was lost when the implications were drawn by policymakers and analysts in other disciplines. In fact, many articles and reports included a caveat such as 'although estimates vary widely ... ', and then went on to discuss worst case scenarios that acted to exaggerate the importance of the military AIDS hypothesis (Mills 2000, Heinecken 2001).

A very important counterfactual argument that needs to be engaged is that militaries have engaged in effective prevention efforts and that this would explain a drop in prevalence rates. There is no doubt that military organisations (especially developed countries, peacekeepers and some developing countries such as Thailand and Uganda), when motivated to take action, were effective at mainstreaming prevention and militaries were sometimes ahead of the national approaches (Healthlink 2002, Sokhey 2004, UN 2009, Lancet 2010). However, the lack of evidence as to the original prevalence rates in militaries and any comprehensive comparative data did not allow this counterfactual to be substantiated.

Why was the military AIDS hypothesis used to support the securitisation of HIV and AIDS?

The most straightforward answer to this question would be that AIDS in military was a serious issue that demanded attention (and resources) (McInnes and Rushton 2010, p. 239). It is clear that securitising any issue has the potential to increase the political commitment to it (Altman 2003, p. 422, McInnes 2006, p. 326). The persistence of the myth could have been as Elbe (2009) notes 'A Noble Lie?' and this is the approach taken by others in highlighting some flawed scientific and policy practice in Asia (Chin 2006), but one that requires much more research to be established. Furthermore, it explains the persistence of the myth up to the late 2000s rather than its birth in politics.

In the context of AIDS exceptionalism the focus on the military AIDS hypothesis that buttressed the broader securitisation of AIDS could be seen as a prudent approach to a potential public health emergency. Elbe (2005) captured this perspective with 'Securitising AIDS, it is hoped, should finally trigger an international political response to the pandemic commensurate with the scale of the humanitarian crisis it bespeaks'. Barnett and Prins note:

> it was a sensible precaution for the UN Security Council to have agreed 1308, which has served to authorise appropriate interventions in uniformed forces... but it must be recognised that the decision to act was based on anecdote and a few more solid, but non public, sources. It was not based... upon a systematic, rigorous and scientific view. (2006)

The potential emergency was more apparent than real.

There was also a geostrategic aspect to the elevation of AIDS as an international security issue. The military AIDS hypothesis took centre stage before the terrorist attacks of 11 September 2001 completely reoriented the security landscape and priorities of policymakers. The issue came to prominence at a time where the agenda was not crowded out by other pressing security concerns. After S11 the need to counter the disproportionate focus being applied to fighting the 'War on Terror' may have contributed to the persistent reliance on the military AIDS hypothesis (Heinecken 2001). The catastrophising that occurs with worst-case scenario planning could as easily be applied to the threat of AIDS as the threat of terror.

Some of the 'securitisation revisionists' did argue that the epidemic was more relevant from a human security perspective than securitisation at the level of national or international security (Becker *et al.* 2008, Elbe 2009). However, the whole point of the military AIDS hypothesis was to elevate the epidemic to be a national and international security concern. It was this conceptual shift that gave the epidemic the prominence that led to the dramatic rise in political (and budgetary/aid) commitment in the early 2000s.

Conclusion

Securitisation and the military AIDS hypothesis that buttressed it, is no longer central to considerations about countering HIV and AIDS. For the purposes of this paper the interesting thing is that the nascent shift is not due to the evidence being recanted. It has been demonstrated that there was never really any robust evidence supporting the military AIDS hypothesis. Therefore we must not ignore the politics of AIDS. Myths can become real and provide potent justifications for international public policy.

In the early 2000s the securitisation of AIDS had become institutionalised in the global approach (UNAIDS) and national responses of developing states and/or peacekeeping states, and many states where the alleged high military infection rates were occurring. Developed states had the resources to prioritise prevention efforts amongst military forces, but an effective international response required the marshalling of political will at the highest levels, significant resources and the institutionalisation of the military AIDS hypothesis through existing and new cooperation between states, intergovernmental organisations and donor agencies. This activity predated the development of an academic consensus on securitisation and evidences the important influence of politics as a driver of public policy noted by Altman (2008a, 2008b) and others.

Holbrooke resigned shortly after changing the international security landscape by elevating AIDS through Resolution 1308. The close relationship between the USA and UN soured over the war in Iraq. The agenda became full with other priorities, namely dealing with the war on terror. So the political constituency supporting securitisation dissipated. On the academic side, McInnes and Rushton (2010) have convincingly argued that the measured response from revisionist academics and practitioners was also influential, especially within the Security Council (Rushton 2010).

More complex connections between AIDS and security were still posited and the prescription among securitisation revisionists was not to reduce resources to dealing with the epidemic, but rather to refocus on a more nuanced response. However, bursting the securitisation bubble may have had unintended consequences for attempts to attract and maintain funding. This has implications in the current environment whereby political leadership has changed, competing priorities (such as climate change) have gained emphasis, and economic crisis is gripping the global economy.

The military AIDS hypothesis is a narrow and specific form of securitisation that sits alongside other perspectives developed during the 1990s and 2000s that securitised AIDS. As such this article provides one means of reviewing the evidence and argument that buttressed the securitisation of AIDS trend. Other perspectives, such as the focus on economic malaise or collapse, state fragility, etc. have been similarly influential in bringing AIDS to centre stage and may not fit the dynamic being reviewed here. That is, they may have a firmer basis in evidence. That said, even these issues, such as the links between state fragility and the epidemic, have also come under sustained scrutiny and criticism. The work of the AIDS Security and Conflict Initiative (ASCI) epitomises this new approach. ASCI's research reports and numerous studies published under its auspices directly challenged the basis for securitisation by targeting the AIDS hypothesis; Sato (2008) noted 'HIV/AIDS is undoubtedly a threat to individual security, but the notion that it risks national defense, and further, international security, is unwarranted' (O'Keefe 2008, ASCI 2009).

This is a classic outcome of securitisation; an endearing argument with catastrophic implications is challenged by reality, but the impact of catastrophising it drowned out the words of caution. It would have been truly shocking if the oft quoted statistic that 40–60% of the Angolan armed forces were HIV positive was true, but it seems that the figures or estimates and the basis for making these estimates was opaque.

There has been a backlash against securitisation, but not necessarily due to the shaky foundations on which it was based. There is growing concern among academics and practitioners that AIDS exceptionalism may have had it's time and place and may have become counterproductive (or an alternative reading would be that it has always been a misplaced focus) (Smith and Whiteside 2010). There is donor fatigue and signs that funding has dropped off (Kaiser Foundation/ UNAIDS 2011) but the epidemic is still the globe's most significant public health challenge.

Thus the aim is to bring the epidemic back into to mainstream discussions of international public health issues so that the epidemic attracts resources. Smith and Whiteside (2010) argue cogently that securitisation rose when ART and other factors made AIDS exceptionalism in developed countries redundant. In the late 1990s the emphasis shifted to developing countries and securitisation was born as a seemingly reasonable justification for a dramatic expansion in efforts to combat HIV and AIDS. Now, global efforts to combat the epidemic face another challenge and securitisation is no longer the answer, and it is clear that there are great risks if politics drives the next stage in the response to the epidemic.

Acknowledgements

The author thanks the editors, Kent Buse and Dennis Altman, and two anonymous reviewers for their constructive criticisms. The author also thanks Molly Anggo for research assistance.

Note

1. As noted earlier, this article relied on information on the public record and does not seek to comment on the existence or accuracy of prevalence statistics produced by militaries but not released for peer review.

References

AIDS Security and Conflict Initiative (ASCI), 2009. *HIV/AIDS, security and conflict: new realities, new responses*. The Hague, Netherlands: ASCI.

Altman, D., 2003. AIDS and security. *International Relations*, 17 (4), 417–427.

Altman, D., 2008a. State fragility, human security and HIV. In: M. Foller and H. Thorn, eds. *The politics of AIDS: globalization, the state and civil society*. Basingstoke: Palgrave.

Altman, D., 2008b. *The political dimensions of responses to HIV/AIDS in Southeast Asia*. The Hague, Netherlands: ASCI, Research Report 5, April.

Anan, K., 2000. *Address to security council, secretary-general says fight against AIDS in Africa immediate priority in global effort against disease*. Press release. New York: United Nations, 6 January.

van den Assum, L. and Rajbhandari, N., 2005. *Towards a UNAIDS framework agenda for AIDS and security*. Geneva: UNAIDS.

Barnett, T. and Prins, G., 2006. HIV/AIDS and security: fact, fiction and evidence – a report to UNAIDS. *International Security*, 82 (2), 359–368.

Bazergan, R., 2003. Intervention and intercourse: HIV/AIDS and peacekeepers. *Conflict, Security and Development*, 3 (1), 27–51, April.

Bazergan, R., 2004. *HIV/AIDS: policies and programs for blue helmets*. Pretoria: Institute for Security Studies, ISS Paper 96, November.

Becker, J., Theodosis, C., and Kulkarni, R., 2008. HIV/AIDS, conflict and security in Africa: rethinking relationships. *Journal of the International AIDS Society*, 11 (3), 1–7.

Bing, E., 2005. Protecting our militaries: a systemic literature review of military HIV/AIDS prevention programs world-wide. *MilMed*, 170 (10), 886–897.

Carballo, M., et al., 2002. *HIV/AIDS and security*. Geneva: International Centre for Migration and Health.

Central Intelligence Agency (CIA), 1987. *Sub-Saharan Africa: implications of the AIDS pandemic*. Washington, DC: CIA (declassified in 2001).

Centre for Conflict Resolution, 2005. *HIV/AIDS and human security: an agenda for Africa*. Seminar Report. Addis Ababa: Centre for Conflict Resolution, September.

Chalk, P., 2001. Pandemic threats to security. In: M. Hansen and W. Tow, eds. *International relations in the new century*. Melbourne: Oxford University Press.

Chen, L., et al., eds., 2003. *Global health challenges for human security*. Cambridge, MA: Harvard University Press.

Chin, J., 2006. *The AIDS pandemic*. Oxford: Radcliffe.

Civil Military Alliance to Combat HIV and AIDS, various years. *Alliance Newsletter*. Hanover: Civil Military Alliance to Combat HIV and AIDS.

Conflict, Security & Development Group, 2000. *Bulletin*, 7, 1–4.

David, M., 2001. Rubber helmets: the certain pitfalls marshaling (SIC) security council resources to combat AIDS in Africa. *Human Rights Quarterly*, 23 (3), 560–582.

Department of Defense HIV/AIDS Prevention Program (DHAAP), 2005. *The first four years: a synopsis of the global effort*. San Diego, CA: DHAAP.

Department of Defense HIV/AIDS Prevention Program (DHAAP), 2009. *2008 Annual Report*, March. San Diego: DHAAP.

Dietrich, J., 2007. The politics of PEPFAR: the president's emergency plan for AIDS relief. *Ethics and International Affairs*, 21 (3), 277–292, Fall.

Dupont, A., 2001a. *East Asia imperilled: transnational challenges to security*. Cambridge: Cambridge University Press.

Dupont, A., 2001b. HIV/AIDS: a major international security issue. *Asia Pacific Ministerial Meeting 9–10 October*, Melbourne.

Eberstadt, N., 2002. The future of AIDS. *Foreign Affairs*, 81 (6), 22–45.

Economic Commission for Africa, 2000. *Leadership at all levels to overcome HIV/AIDS*. Addis Ababa: Economic Commission for Africa, December.

Elbe, S., 2002. HIV/AIDS and the changing landscape of war in Africa. *International Security*, 27 (2), 159–177.

Elbe, S., 2003. *Strategic implications of HIV/AIDS*. Adelphi Paper. Oxford: Oxford University Press.

Elbe, S., 2005. AIDS, security, biopolitics. *International Relations*, 19 (4), 403–419.

Elbe, S., 2006. Should AIDS be securitised? The ethical dilemmas of linking HIV/AIDS and security. *International Studies Quarterly*, 50 (1), 119–144.

Elbe, S., 2009. *Virus alert: security, governmentality, and the AIDS epidemic*. New York: Columbia University Press.

Fitzsimons, D. and Whiteside, A., 1992. The AIDS epidemic: economic, political and security implications. *Conflict Studies*, 271, 1–37.

Foreman, M., 2002. *HIV/AIDS infection in the military*. London: Healthlink.

Fourie, P. and Schonteich, M., 2001. Africa's new security threat: HIV/AIDS and human security in Southern Africa. *African Defence Review*, 10 (1), 29–44.

Garrett, L., 2005. *HIV and national security: where are the links?* New York: Council on Foreign Relations, Report.

Gore, A., 2000. *Statement in the security council on AIDS in Africa*. Washington, DC: White House, Office of the Vice President, 10 January.

Goyer, K., 2001. HIV and political instability in sub-Saharan Africa. *AIDS and Africa*, 12 (1), 13 and 16.

Hankins, C., et al., 2002. Transmission and prevention of HIV and sexually transmitted infections in war settings: implications for current and future armed conflicts. *AIDS*, 16 (17), 2245–2252.

Harker, J., 2001. *HIV-AIDS and the security sector in Canada: a threat to Canada*. Commentary No. 80, 26 September. Canadian Security Intelligence Service, 6–7.

Healthlink, 2002. *Combat AIDS: HIV and the world's armed forces*. London: Healthlink.

Heinecken, L., 2001. Living in terror: the looming security threat to Southern Africa. *African Security Review*, 10 (4), 6–17.

Heinecken, L., 2003. Facing a merciless enemy: HIV/AIDS and the South African armed forces. *Armed Forces and Society*, 29 (2), 281–300, Winter.

Hsu, L., 2001. *HIV subverts national security*. Bangkok: UNDP South East Asia HIV and Development Report, August.

Inter Agency Standing Committee (IASC), 2004. *Guidelines for HIV/AIDS interventions in emergency settings*. Geneva: IASC.

Kaiser Foundation/UNAIDS, 2011. *Financing the response to AIDS in low- and middle-income countries: international assistance from the G8, European Commission and other donor governments in 2010*. Geneva: Kaiser Foundation/UNAIDS, August.

Kingma, S., 1996. *AIDS prevention in military populations: learning the lessons from history*. Civil-Military Alliance to Combat HIV and AIDS, Occasional Paper Series, no. 2.

Lancet, 2010. The art of medicine: HIV/AIDS and the challenges of security and conflict. *Lancet*, 375 (9708), 22–23.

Lowicki-Zucca, M., Karmin, S., and Dehne, K.-L., 2009. HIV among peacekeepers and its likely impact on prevalence on host countries' HIV epidemics. *International Peacekeeping*, 16 (3), 352–363.

McInnes, C., 2006. HIV/AIDS and security. *International Affairs*, 82 (2), 315–326.

McInnes, C., 2009. Conflict, HIV and AIDS: a new dynamic in warfare? *Global Change, Peace and Security*, 21 (1), 99–114.

McInnes, C., 2011. HIV, AIDS and conflict in Africa: why isn't it (even) worse? *Review of International Studies*, 37 (2), 485–509.

McInnes, C. and Rushton, S., 2010. HIV, AIDS and security: where are we now? *International Affairs*, 86 (1), 225–245.

Mills, G., 2000. AIDS and the South African military: timeworn cliché or timebomb? Konrad Adenauer Stiftung Occasional Papers, St Augustin, Germany, June, 67–73.

National Intelligence Council (NIC), 2000. *The global infectious disease threat and its implications for the United States*. Washington, DC: NIC, January.

NIC, 2008. *Strategic implications of global health*. Washington, DC: NIC.

O'Keefe, M., 2008. *State fragility and AIDS in the South Pacific*. The Hague, Netherlands: AIDS, Security and Conflict Institute (ASCI), ASCI Research Report No. 9.

O'Keefe, M., 2011. Contextualising the AIDS epidemic in the South Pacific: orthodoxies, estimates and evidence. *Australian Journal of International Affairs*, 65 (2), 185–202.

Ogba, L., 1989. Violence, conflict and health in Africa. *Social Sciences Medicine*, 28 (7), 649–657.

Ostergard, R., 2002. Politics in the hot zone: AIDS and national security in Africa. *Third World Quarterly*, 23 (2), 333–350.

Oumar, B., et al., 2008. HIV/AIDS in African militaries: an ecological analysis. *Medicine, Conflict and Survival*, 24 (2), 88–100.

Rushton, S., 2010. AIDS and international security in the United Nations System. *Health Policy and Planning*, 25 (6), 495–504.

Sarin, R., 2003. A new security threat: HIV/AIDS in the military. *Worldwatch*, 16 (2), 17–22.

Sato, A., 2008. *Is HIV/AIDS a threat to security in fragile states?* The Hague, Netherlands: ASCI.

Save the Children, 2002. *HIV and conflict: a double emergency*. London: Save the Children.

Schneider, M. and Moodie, M., 2002. *The destabilizing impacts of HIV/AIDS*. Washington, DC: CSIS HIV/AIDS Task Force, May.

Singer, P., 2002. AIDS and international security. *Survival*, 44 (1), 145–158.

Smith, J. and Whiteside, A., 2010. The history of AIDS exceptionalism. *Journal of the International AIDS Society*, 13 (47), 1–8.

Sokhey, T., 2004. *Mainstreaming HIV prevention in the military: a case study from Cambodia*. Bangkok: UNDP South East Asia HIV and Development Programme.

Speigel, P., *et al.*, 2007. Prevalence of HIV infection in conflict-affected and displaced people in seven sub-Saharan African countries: a systematic review. *Lancet*, 369 (9580), 2187–2195.

Tripodi, P., *et al.*, 2001. The global impact of HIV/AIDS on peace support operations. *International Peacekeeping*, 9 (3), 51–66.

UN, 2000. *UNSC, resolution 1308 (2000), adopted by the security council at its 4172nd meeting, 17 July 2000*. New York: United Nations.

UN, 2001. *UNSC, 4259th meeting*, 19 January 2001, S/PV.4259. New York: United Nations.

UN, 2009. *UN pre-deployment training (PDT) standards*. Core PDT materials. 1st ed. New York: United Nations.

UNAIDS, 1998. *AIDS and the military: UNAIDS point of view*. New York: UNAIDS.

UN General Assembly, 2001. *Declaration of commitment on HIV/AIDS*. New York: United Nations, June.

de Waal, A., 2002. Fucking soldiers. *Index on censorship*, 31 (4), 87–92.

Whiteside, A., de Waal, A., and Gebre-Tensae, T., 2006. AIDS, security and the military in Africa: a sober reappraisal. *African Affairs*, 105 (419), 201–218.

Williams, M., 2003. Words, images, enemies: securitization and international politics. *International Studies Quarterly*, 47 (4), 511–531.

Yeager, R., *et al.*, 2000. International military human immunodeficiency virus/acquired immunodeficiency syndrome politics and programs: strengths and limitations of current practice. *Military Medicine: International Journal of AMSUS*, 156 (2), 81–92.

AIDS hyper-epidemics and social resilience: theorising the political

Pieter Fourie and Maj-Lis Follér

AIDS has been the most political pandemic in the world for 30 years, and yet political science has viewed it in a mostly descriptive, compartmentalised and theoretically neglectful way. There have been many theories of AIDS, but very little AIDS theory that is informed by politics. This deficit of theory seems to be intellectually counter-intuitive, but may be the result of an epistemic community which is often erroneously constructed as monolithic; its pursuits are deeply informed by funding priorities which favour phenomena with more tangible, short-term results; the incremental biomedical 'good practice' responses in some instances crowd out what is perceived as the luxury of deeper, systemic reflection. This article argues that a focus on socio-political resilience can be useful to galvanise political scientific theorising of AIDS. As a heuristic filter, resilience may be useful to advance social science's analytical narrative regarding the pandemic beyond the negative, to identify and capitalise on the lessons and transformational potential of AIDS and other long-wave shocks.

Introduction

For the most part, political science was late in responding to the global AIDS pandemic, particularly in the context of hyper-epidemics.[1] However, once the discipline and its various constituencies turned their attention to the reality and challenges of the pandemic, it moved to conceptualise aspects of AIDS into neat but by now quite dated epistemic boxes.

Some of these categories include research focusing broadly on impact (this is often sectoral or case study work) (e.g. Kaiser Family Foundation 2007); studies reflecting on the response of specific (mostly domestic/national) political constituencies, particularly in hyper-epidemics (e.g. Strand *et al.* 2004); studies describing transnational, non-state responses, mainly an evolving global AIDS civil society (e.g. Friedman and Mottiar 2005); public administrative and cognate disciplines, which are particularly interested in the impact of AIDS on democratic process and 'good' governance practices (taking a chiefly institutionalist approach) (e.g. Chirambo 2006); area/comparative approaches (mostly case studies) (e.g. Seckinelgin 2008), and security studies (e.g. Elbe 2009), which was a particularly lucrative area of study in the years following the 9/11 attacks in the USA.

There has been surprisingly little political science scholarship on the *transformational* potential of the pandemic (e.g. Sidibé *et al.* 2010). Thus far, political science mostly seems to have shied away from AIDS as a truly long-wave event, with little theorising of the pandemic in post-Westphalian or non-state terms.

In this article we are specifically interested in the pandemic as a political (i.e. power- and agency-shifting) opportunity for socio-cultural innovation and resilience. The epidemic challenges the political status quo of not only the private sphere (in terms of gender relations, for instance), but also more broadly where power is located socially as well as globally. For instance, during the past decade the global pandemic has done much to alter conceptions of and indeed actual international law governing intellectual property, it has mobilised the establishment and funding of vast new multilateral institutions, and it has demanded significant shifts in the governance and flow of overseas development assistance.

Political science has identified and analysed these recent shifts in the rules and institutions that govern the *impact* of AIDS globally, but it has not produced a significant body of theory to understand the full political manifestations of the epidemic, or responses to it. This article focuses on AIDS and the theme of resilience – in particular how resilience may be useful to reinvigorate political scientific theorising of AIDS and other long-wave events. Frustratingly, resilience Studies have almost exclusively focused on the natural sciences, building theory regarding the systemic, long-term impact of natural disasters. Punctuated Equilibrium (Colgan *et al.* 2011), Evolutionary Theory (Rostow 1960) and Systems Theory (Easton 1965) are other examples of natural scientific theories that are sometimes transferred to the social sciences. There is a real opportunity for a political scientific exploration of resilience in the context of AIDS – as a natural, socio-cultural and political phenomenon.

Our analysis is structured as follows: first we introduce the concept of 'resilience', exploring ways in which it can be made applicable to the context of human society in addition to its orthodox focus on the biological, natural world. Second, we briefly review the transformative power of epidemics in human history, before, in the third instance, identifying some tentative ways in which the ongoing AIDS pandemic, as a long-wave event, may be changing societies, channelling understandings of 'impact' in both the negative sense, but also constructively. Political science has been remiss in contributing to this latter narrative, but applying the filter of social resilience might enable it to recalibrate its body of theory on AIDS and other cross-generational events.

Understanding 'resilience', politically

On 18 August 2010 the UN Office for the Coordination of Humanitarian Affairs' online news service, *IRIN News*, reported that

> [i]ncreasing strains on a century-old, five-nation southern African customs union is raising questions as to whether the sovereignty of its poorest members – Lesotho and Swaziland – is sustainable, considering their burden of HIV/AIDS and the global economic slowdown...

This report came within weeks of an earlier one, in Britain's *Observer* newspaper, which on 6 June 2010 reported that '[t]housands of people in the impoverished Commonwealth kingdom of Lesotho have asked South Africa [...] to annex their state because it has been bankrupted by the HIV pandemic' (Smith 2010, p. 11).

Just more than one in four Swazi nationals aged 15–49 years are living with HIV; at 26.1%, this is the world's highest national adult prevalence. In Lesotho there is a 23.2% national HIV infection rate, and in nearby Botswana the level is slightly higher, at 24.6%, whilst Namibia as well as the dominant state in the region, South Africa, each have adult prevalence levels of around 20%. Left untreated, these countries would stand to lose at least one in four or one in five adults to AIDS during the next decade.

Tragic as this reality is, individual AIDS watchers and governments have known about these numbers and such consequences for some years, and yet AIDS fatigue has started to set in. The burden of other, neglected diseases and the impact of the ongoing global financial crisis are hitting hard, with donor support for AIDS programmes slipping away. This does not bode well for a sustained rollout of the drugs needed to keep the impact of the AIDS pandemic at bay.

Compounding the personal tragedies being played out in homes and communities in the context of mature AIDS epidemics, the two news reports quoted above draw attention to the potential for an additional, insidious and eminently political consequence of the pandemic: institutional, multilateral and eventual state failure – these countries are in danger of collapsing.[2]

Of course, 'collapse', or deep, systemic (and often sudden) change is not a new phenomenon in the evolution and study of societies and political organisations. Entire civilisations have changed fundamentally: the Roman, Greek, Egyptian, Mayan and Inca empires of old have all made way for more modern, state-based regimes, and according to the conservative historian, Ferguson (2010), even the American empire is exhibiting some classic symptoms of 'imperial overstretch' – fiscal overspending, uncontrolled deficits – and is in danger of eventual collapse.

Epidemics are often mentioned as being some of the key contributors to such collapse and regime change at scale. Increasingly, over the last two decades, analyses of the 'impact' of AIDS usually centre on how the pandemic erodes households' and societies' ability to care for themselves, to sustain economic growth, and to distribute the benefits of such growth in an equitable manner. In particular, since the terrorist attacks in the USA on 11 September 2001, a narrative of securitisation has come to dominate much of the political science literature on AIDS. The UN Security Council in 2000 already declared AIDS a threat to national security globally, eroding the ability of states to maintain their monopoly on violence, possibly even presaging international conflicts as well as civil wars, and state collapse.

We acknowledge but wish to move beyond these narratives of doom. Surely 'impact' does not in all instances only equate with a sense of creeping decay, erosion, destruction and death? Can AIDS and other health threats not also lead to socio-political innovation, adaptation and positive social change? In asking these questions, we wish to make it clear that at the individual, family and household levels, AIDS and other poverty-driven health threats are unmitigated disasters; we do not agree with, nor do we wish to give voice to the position of either those neo-Malthusian racists or the Social Darwinian 'survival of the fittest' types who suggest that natural disasters and disease are simply nature's way of taking care of overpopulation. We are not suggesting that the morbidity and the mortality associated with health disasters are a good thing.

In every tragedy there is scope for learning, innovation and change; 'impact', however bad it is, always begets victors as well as losers, survivors as well as victims. We are interested in why some societies and states are more resilient than others to the impact and consequences of external shocks. Is it the way in which they are governed? Are some cultural beliefs and practices more constructive in terms of the kinds of responses that they facilitate in the face of systemic shocks? Can the nascent field of 'resilience thinking' – even though it tends to focus on natural shocks in biological systems, rather than looking at disasters in socio-human ecological contexts – help political and other social scientists to make sense of why and how some societies are sustainable and responsive to threats, rather than collapsing?

Is it possible to find political scientific foundations for socio-economic resilience?

According to Walker and Salt (2006, p. 1) resilience refers to 'the ability of a system to absorb disturbance and still retain its basic function and structure'. They later paraphrase this definition, saying that '[r]esilience is the capacity of a system to absorb disturbance without shifting to another regime' (Walker and Salt 2006, p. 37). Clearly, the concept is closely related to notions of sustainable development, learning, the emergence of novelty, creativity and adaptability, as well as the ability of a society or a natural system to regenerate. Holling *et al.* (2002, p. 5) add to this that resilience thinking '... must of necessity transcend boundaries of scale and discipline. It must be capable of organising our understanding of economic, ecological and institutional systems'.

At the heart of resilience thinking is the notion of adaptability, and an embrace of change. Stasis in the face of a systemic challenge or a shock to any system means destruction and regression, whereas dynamism and adaptability are viewed as progressive and constructive. Holling and Gunderson (2002, p. 27) warn that there are two grand popular notions regarding resilience: the first one emphasises efficiency, control, constancy and predictability, but these attributes do not allow for sustainability in the long run, as they sit uneasily with 'real' resilience, which does not fear unpredictability. In order to be sustainable, the second, authentic notion of resilience must dominate: societies or any 'regime' (to use the phrase applied by resilience thinkers) must embrace challenge, movement and adaptability, as the alternative is complacency and atrophy.

Other concepts applied in resilience thinking include 'thresholds' and 'feedback loops'. The idea of thresholds is well-established, of course, especially since the notion of 'tipping points' was popularised by Gladwell (2000) in his book *The Tipping Point: How Little Things Can Make a Big Difference*, and the appearance of popular management material such as Ball's (2004) *Critical Mass: How One Thing Leads to Another*. Thresholds are important in many fields of study, in – as well as outside of – quantitative and natural sciences: economists revere gross domestic product and other threshold metrics, political scientists often embrace rational choice descriptors, and in social epidemiology we now know that a CD4 count below 350 per measure of blood is the clinical threshold of AIDS-related complex (or 'full-blown AIDS'), which the World Health Organization uses as its threshold indicator for treatment initiation with anti-retroviral drugs.

In resilience thinking, though, thresholds are important in the sense that they are the markers of movement within a system, from one regime to another. In other words, if a society or a system can absorb a shock successfully, its distance from tipping points or thresholds indicating change is also a good indicator of how imperilled it is by such a shock, and of how resilient it was to that shock. For instance, *Foreign Policy* and *The Fund for Peace* have conceptualised a methodology (see www.foreignpolicy.com/failedstates) which also contain an early warning system of possible collapse amongst weak/fragile states. Some of the elements of this early warning system include indices of risk, and combinations of risk co-factors could presage eventual state disintegration. As events develop the model is refined, with threshold limits and tipping points constantly being recalibrated and developed as time goes on.

A 'feedback loop', on the other hand, refers to systems of nature which, according to resilience thinking, usually proceed through recurring cycles consisting of four phases: rapid growth, conservation, release and reorganisation: '[t]he manner in which the system behaves is different from one phase to the next with changes in the strength of the system's internal connections, its flexibility, and its resilience' (Walker and Salt 2006, p. 75). This dynamic system is referred to as the 'adaptive cycle', and is usually presented as in Figure 1.

In our conception of the adaptive cycle, the 'release' phase represents a shock or a challenge to how a regime or a system of any kind operates. As resilience thinkers tend to come from the natural sciences, the release cycle often refers to something like a large-scale tsunami, or a potentially devastating fire in a rainforest, but for our purposes, the AIDS pandemic can also be viewed as such a systemic shock. The latter destroys some of the reserves that a system has accumulated, but if it is responsive to the release, reorganisation is possible, so that collapse does not ultimately happen, but rather the growth or exploitation phase is able to continue.

In societies or systems where there is no conservation of surplus production, little embrace of insights from history and no culture of proactively adapting to factors that upset the status quo, the release/shock phase can lead to the destruction of that particular regime. In the context of health shocks, the impact of AIDS in Swaziland and Lesotho as described above has been such that those regimes are now reported to be unable to be self-sustaining: individuals,

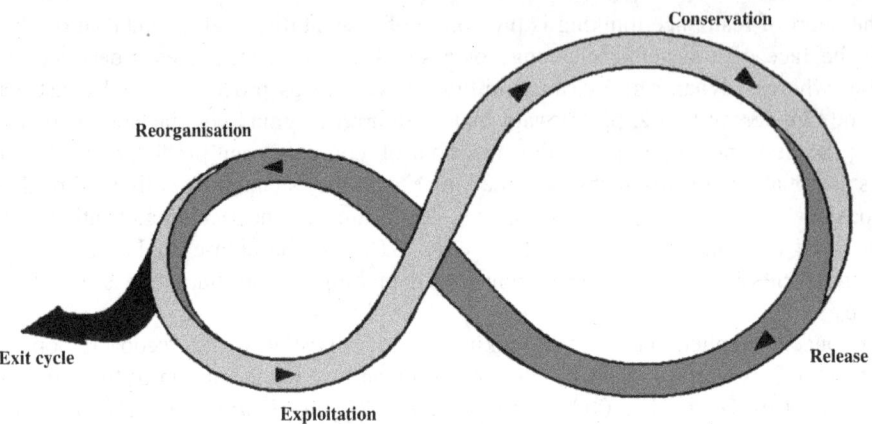

Figure 1. The 'adaptive cycle' in resilience thinking (Holling and Gunderson 2002).

households, families and ultimately the state are put under such pressure that their very existence is compromised. This is the AIDS 'doom' narrative that we identified earlier.

Instead, we are interested in the other side of that coin: what would it take for a society that is being threatened by a mature AIDS pandemic to move successfully from the release phase to reorganisation? Walker and Salt (2006, pp. 122–124) provide some guidance in response to such a question. In terms of policy-making (useful for political science as well as for national policy-makers) which is responsive to and that applies the principles of resilience thinking in the context of HIV and AIDS, the following insights are key:

- Ecosystems and social systems cannot and should not be managed in isolation, for that would ignore the feedback loops between them, stifling adaptability (the natural/biological is eminently political). Viewing the AIDS epidemic as something abstract and discreet from the society that it affects is not useful.
- It is important to get a sense of the threshold limits that apply in a specific context, in order to enable change in good time. Political 'best practice', also in terms of responses to AIDS, is contingent rather than universal. For instance, a strong public health intervention which shuns human rights but enables effective interventions might work in a specific context at a certain time along that epidemic's trajectory (e.g. Cuba in the 1980s), but such a response might not be appropriate and actually counterproductive in, for instance, Swaziland in the mid-1990s.
- It is important to be aware of the scale at which one is planning for a shock to the system. One should include household-level planning as well as more macro-, social-level planning and policy-making.
- Identify possible alternate regimes for the system (political analysis should be deductive rather than inductive).
- Identify key points for intervention (this is important for policy-making, risk assessment and planning).
- Devise subsidies *for* change, rather than subsidies *not to* change – and build redundancies into planning. What lessons can be heeded from the impact of the epidemic in a specific context?
- Invest in building adaptability and promote (do not hinder) experimentation and learning.
- Design or modify existing governance structures. For instance, (1) consider alternatives to existing electoral and Parliamentary representative systems which allow for greater

redundancy amongst elected representatives, and (2) establish institutions that will remain responsive to the long-term impact of the epidemic.
- Acknowledge that there is a cost to maintaining resilience. The epidemic demands tough choices in determining how resources are allocated, and not everyone will benefit.

Even though Walker and Salt's definition of resilience can apply to both socio-human and bio-natural ecological complexes, the literature on resilience thinking is rather slight on socio-human areas of sustainability, and the key texts on 'resilience thinking' almost exclusively deal with the natural world. Even in the more popular treatment and application of the concept, public intellectuals such as Diamond (2005), in his book *Collapse: How Societies Choose to Fail or Survive*, or Homer-Dixon (2006), in his *The Upside of Down: Catastrophe, Creativity, and the Renewal of Civilisation*, and Tainter (2008), in *The Collapse of Complex Societies*, focus mainly on the human degradation of the biosphere, and how such man-made climate change imperils societies and leads to the fall of civilisations. That said, Holling *et al.* (2002, p. 3) do mention the theme of this article explicitly, emphasising that

> [n]ovel diseases have emerged in socially and ecologically disturbed areas of the world and have spread globally ... The tragedy of AIDS, and it origins, transformation, and dispersion because of land-use and social changes, is a signal of deep and broad changes that will yield further surprises and crises.

Unfortunately such reflection on human societies and their resilience, rather than a focus exclusively on the resilience of the natural world, are few and far between (for a notable exception, see Galaz *et al.* 2010). Walker *et al.* (2006) address this issue in another publication, stating that '[t]he ecological and social domains of social-ecological systems can be addressed in a common conceptual, theoretical, and modelling framework'. Adger (2000, p. 347) agrees, reminding us that '[e]cological and social resilience may be linked through the dependence on ecosystems of communities and their economic activities'. Again, the true meaning and emphasis of 'sustainable development' comes to the fore (Holling 2001), referring to the dual goal of fostering adaptive capabilities and creating opportunities.

Adger (2000, p. 350) suggests that we should focus on 'social resilience' rather than on 'resilience', the latter tending to be related to the natural world and the ecosystem only. In contrast, social resilience is purported to be more sensitive to the interplay between sustainability and human institutions, and (importantly) it is also sensitive to the positive and negative aspects of eminently political elements such as social exclusion, marginalisation, social capital and issues of equity and justice. Marshall and Marshall (2007) further develop the idea of social resilience, suggesting that it should refer closely to societies' perception of risk in approaching change, the ability to plan, learn and reorganise, the ability to cope with change and to building institutions that can enable a society to adapt. In particular, they point to policy change as a key feature of social resilience: if a state or an institution of power is unable to identify and evaluate policy alternatives, allow for policy change as well as the concomitant mobilisation of adequate resources, then a challenge to the regime will lead to its collapse rather than enhancing its sustainability.

The next section addresses the question of whether and how epidemics in history have had political impacts in societies beyond the predictable focus on raised morbidity and mortality levels.

Epidemics and political change in history

From a health perspective, if you live in the developed world and have a regular income, then this is probably the best time in human history to be alive. People in the rich world can now look forward to such long lives that their very longevity has become a key concern – but this is a very recent development. Until Germ Theory became well-established in the late 1800s, and until the take-off in medical science after World War II, life for most people was 'nasty, brutish and short'. In fact, in the decade or so after 1945 there was such a strong faith in the ability of medical technology in general and in antibiotics and vaccines in particular, that the medical community started to speak of a world without any burden of infectious disease. However, since the 1970s a number of old diseases have re-emerged and terrifying epidemics of brand new pathogens have come to mock any utopian notion of life beyond sickness.

History provides good examples and opportunities for natural as well as social scientists to learn about the diseases and epidemics that made us, that created the world in which we live. Epidemics and other significant systemic shocks to past regimes have been powerful determinants of our civilisation today. Then, as now, some societies have faded away, whilst others flourished, managing to maintain and build their resilience. Baker (2007) considers the scale and impact of a number of diseases and epidemics in history:

- The great influenza (Spanish flu) epidemic of 1918–1920 killed between 50 and 100 million people, most of them young. This makes the Spanish flu the most lethal pandemic in known history. Should its mortality be repeated with the contemporary global population, it would kill in excess of 300 million people.
- AIDS has already killed around 30 million people, and an even greater number live with HIV today. The global pandemic is not in decline, with incidence outpacing prevention efforts (even if the rate of new infections has diminished).
- Malaria has been a companion to humans for millennia, and today it kills 2.7 million people every year. Around 3000 children die of malaria every day, and one consequence of climate change will be a surge in malarial infections globally.
- Cholera killed millions in India immediately after it first appeared in Calcutta in 1817, and humans have been unable to stop its spread: it still kills between one and two million children under the age of five every year.
- Smallpox killed as many as five million people during the Antonine Plague of 165–180 AD, and was instrumental in the death of tens of millions of people living in the Americas in the wake of the arrival of Europeans.
- Typhus may have lost the Athenians the war against the Peloponnesian League, led by Sparta. Colossal mortality from typhus also occurred during Napoleon's 1815 retreat from Moscow.

Diseases and epidemics are not simply and exclusively biological phenomena that one can approach by biomedicine and public health interventions alone. As Michel Foucault and others (e.g. Altman 1986, Treichler 1999, Sontag 2002, Barnes 2005, Crawford 2007) remind us, epidemics are political, social and cultural constructs as much as they are natural entities. Robert Hudson (quoted in Hays 2009, p. 3) captures this well, saying that '[d]iseases are not immutable entities but dynamic social constructions that have biographies of their own'. As such, epidemics have the capacity to change the ways in which humans perceive their world, power relations within societies, and the very nature of reality itself. For instance, Germ Theory challenged the very idea that disease is some kind of divine retribution or punishment for collective or individual human vice; tuberculosis continues to challenge notions that the poor and their suffering matter less than the rich and their maladies; cholera revolutionised sanitation and the management of waste and water across multiple societies (Evans 1988).

The Black Death is a particularly good example of a pandemic that had an impact over time, remaking entire societies. It arose in the fourteenth century, with serial peaks of epidemics up until the eighteenth century, and even sporadic outbreaks into the modern era. It is said to have killed 34 million people in Europe alone, with similar numbers in Asia. In terms of impact, change, adaptability and, ultimately, resilience in the context of the Black Death, much has been written about the deep, systemic changes to Western European society that came in the wake of the pandemic.

At the most basic level, there was a fundamental and dramatic change in the demography of European society; it killed between 30% and 60% of everyone in many affected communities. This led to changed conceptions about who was important, how the state could tax the people in its jurisdiction (Cohn 2007), how divisions of labour had to be adapted in order to maintain the production of food and its commerce, and this ultimately challenged and changed the entire European political economy, contributing to the end of feudalism (Cartwright and Biddiss 2006). It also led to the challenging of the authority of the Roman Catholic Church, and a questioning of the power of the priests to banish disease. Such a metaphysical shift in conceptions of the cosmos and causal links between the physical and the metaphysical/supernatural worlds eroded the power of religious workers, and may have led to secularisation across Europe, sparking the spirit of Enlightenment.

Epidemics continue to act as agents of change in contemporary society, in determining how the world works. Infectious disease continues to kill more people than military or civil strife, but it affects the present in other, profound ways also. When humanity is lucky it even holds the promise of constructive introspection, changing the world for the better and increasing societies' moral fortitude and physical resilience. For instance, improved instruments and global institutions have been put in place to ensure a timely response to epidemics. The World Health Organization was established after World War II and co-ordinates early epidemic detection mechanisms across the world; its International Health Regulations provide important criteria for the management of and general responsiveness to the outbreak of biological threats. Cooper and Kirton (2008) hail these *innovations* (an important word in resilience thinking) as progress in the human management and political governance of disease globally.

Less directly, but maybe even more importantly, there have been some dramatic cultural advances in human conceptions of disease and epidemics. Contemporary pathogens challenge societies to reflect on what it means to be a good and caring global community, who should care for those who are unable to afford life-saving medical technologies, how one should think about the political control of biotechnologies, and how they are regulated (Fukuyama 2003). According to McMichael (2004, p. 1052)

> ... we are living through [...a] great historical transition. This time scale is global and changes are occurring on many fronts. The spread and increased lability of various infectious diseases, new and old, reflect the impacts of demographic, environmental, social, technological and other rapid changes in human ecology. [... I]t underscores how configurations of social and environmental influences change.

Applying a human ecological approach to contemporary epidemics, Wilson (1995) emphasises that it is critical for societies to remain responsive and adaptable to the emergence and impact of pandemics. In order to do so, she argues that Western societies and states need to move beyond too strict and exclusive a focus on surveillance. This is a timely warning, as surveillance has tended to become the be all and end all of a securitised response to epidemics, especially after 9/11.

Her point is not that surveillance in itself is a bad thing – it is critically important and integrated with the International Health Regulations, for instance, which 'aim is to help the international community prevent and respond to acute public health risks that have the potential to cross borders and threaten people worldwide' (WHO 2012). Surveillance should not become a goal in itself; it should be part of a larger process of which the overall aim is to improve the human condition and to remain responsive to the challenges posed by pathogens and other systemic shocks.

Wilson (1995) suggests that societies should apprehend infectious diseases in their evolutionary and ecological context, and *respond to that context* rather than only formulating short-term responses to recently surveyed outbreaks. Such a response is political, as it will only be possible if we recognise the links between population growth, climatic and environmental change, global migration and human health and security; develop databases that combine information about climate, demography, population movements, and diseases in humans, animals and plants; identify markers for regions or populations at high risk of epidemic disease so that we can intervene to reduce the impact of disease; continue efforts to slow population growth; take steps to reduce mass migration and displacement of populations; reduce consumption and pay more attention to land use and production and disposal of toxins and chemicals; take a broader view and longer time frame when analysing the potential impact of interventions; view human life as part of a constantly evolving biosphere. Each of these activities imply political interpretations and political decisions taken by individuals and political bodies who have the power to act; as Michel Foucault and Sontag (2003) remind us, the very act of observing/surveillance and interpretation is political.

The lessons or 'gifts' of disasters and epidemics in particular seem clear enough when one looks closely, and most particularly when one applies resilience thinking, with a different time frame in mind. Most recently, AIDS has become a new galvaniser of change.

AIDS and deep, systemic change

It is significant that Wilson emphasises the importance of using a longer time frame when planning for the impact of epidemics and interventions, as the most lethal epidemics quite counterintuitively tend to be those that evolve slowly, and sometimes invisibly. Examples include the Black Death, which was active and killing people over centuries, and AIDS, which, according to Prof. Roy Anderson of Imperial College, London, could have an epidemic curve of 130 years (De Waal and Whiteside 2006). Regular political analyses of the impact of epidemics tend to use the language of securitisation, which is keen to underscore the imminent peril and the severity of the pandemic threats. Securitisation is a useful strategy for governments and societies to respond to threats, as it creates a sense of crisis, and a spirit of mobilisation: public health interventions can be activated; interfering laws, rules and regulations can be suspended to enable rapid intervention; institutions, budgets and manpower can be provided to combat the initial spread of the epidemic, and short-term measures can be put in place.

AIDS is different. It is a *lentivirus*, which means that, epidemiologically, it moves slowly, takes its time to infect a large cohort of people within society, and even once infection has taken place, it takes many years to kill. This means that the AIDS pandemic, rather than exhibiting immediate and dramatic impacts, is a 'long-wave event', which unfolds over an extended period of time.

Long-wave events, whether they are pandemics, or climate change, or systemic changes in the global political economy, share a number of characteristics (Barnett 2006, pp. 302–303): it is unclear when they start; by the time governments or societies are aware of their existence, it is difficult to actually do anything about their evolution; building strategies to neutralise their negative impacts takes time, and requires interventions that would address the long term (this is a challenge to many governments, given that elected officials tend to be in office for relatively short periods of time); managing their consequences makes novel demands, requires innovation, and there are few precedents to shine a light on the path towards resilience; dealing with them lies beyond what single governments and administrations can do; the contemporary culture of securitising pandemics and other threats is anachronous in the context of long-wave events, as they often require deep, systemic responses and change, rather than short-term thinking and crisis interventions.

The long-wave nature of the AIDS pandemic makes it a particular challenge to address by governments and other institutions of power. The securitisation of any issue is useful in that it creates an immediate sense of danger, galvanises political will and thus enabling the rapid mobilisation of human and material resources. Given the very long-wave nature of the AIDS pandemic, political science's use of securitisation as a lens to understand HIV has simply not been very useful to either describe the impact of AIDS, or to suggest appropriate policy responses. Resilience thinking is geared towards long-term planning and thus it could be instructive in identifying positive feedback loops to enable planning and strategising that are more appropriate to the timescale of the event. Thirty years after AIDS first made newspaper headlines, resilience thinking is yet to make a constructive contribution to planning for its impact. Instead, thus far there has been a lot of reactive policy-making at both national and global/multilateral levels. These policies tend to fall into the short-termism trap usually associated with dramatic and rapidly spreading epidemics, and has created significant AIDS fatigue in governments (Lyman and Wittels 2010), in the global donor community (Over 2009), as well as in communities affected by the virus. At the same time, it can also be said that on one level the HIV response has been attempting to shift the norms and the behaviours of two generations, for example, to use condoms, and to provide greater autonomy over one's (women's, in particular) bodies; these are challenging goals, but they have a long-term rather than a short-term focus.

Short-term planning and a reactive mindset have led to two major misunderstandings. The first relates to the perception of AIDS as a blanket threat to the security and sustainability of states. Over the last decade in particular, AIDS watchers have sought to demonstrate that the pandemic is eroding states' ability to achieve and sustain adequate levels of economic growth, to distribute the benefits of that growth in an equitable manner, to maintain a monopoly on violence in societies where huge numbers of people are already living with HIV, and that the epidemic is undermining democratic governance.

As demonstrated elsewhere (De Waal 2006, Fourie 2009), though, there simply is not sufficient evidence to suggest that AIDS is leading to state collapse – for the moment. Armies have not mutinied, wars have not started and there is no eruption of crime in societies where AIDS has reached hyper-epidemic proportions. There is also no evidence to suggest that the pandemic is undermining democratic practice, or that it has led to the collapse of entire economic sectors. There are only three instances that we are aware of where a direct link has been drawn between a mature AIDS epidemic, and any great assault on state sovereignty, as well as social sustainability: the two reports cited earlier, and a study by the World Bank (Bell et al. 2006) which speculates (but cannot prove) that the generational effect of AIDS on economic growth in South Africa will be such that the country will collapse a few decades hence.

The second major point of confusion that short-termism (i.e. non-resilience thinking) constitutes the primary strategy to combat the pandemic. Many donor organisations, national governments and multilateral institutions have been so concerned with the neutralisation of the supposed security threats from AIDS, as well as so busy focusing on the discovery of quick fix medical technological solutions to the pandemic, that some of the most fundamental, intractable and systemic challenges associated with AIDS have been neglected. (We do not wish to discount the work of many agencies on prevention in particular: UNAIDS' prevention evolution focuses not only on combination prevention but takes an overtly political approach (UNAIDS 2010).

The point is that so much energy and so many resources have gone into attempts to *treat* AIDS (mainly through the development and dissemination of anti-retroviral drugs), that only lip-service is paid to the most long-lasting and sustainable response to the pandemic: effective *prevention*, with a focus on behaviour change and social mobilisation (Epstein 2007). Without such a shift in focus, as well as the deep socio-cultural change that this would require over time, Over (2010) warns that a true 'AIDS transition' – moving to a point where incidence drops and eventually reduces aggregate prevalence levels – would remain impossible.

In order to make the fantasy a reality, AIDS thought leaders and policy-makers need to start applying resilience thinking, think systemically, and use a longer time horizon to work towards sustainable change. We need to identify and to build upon the positive social innovation and changes that AIDS can enable. In the parlance of social resilience, one of the key 'gifts' of the AIDS pandemic could be the feedback loops, those lessons learnt about how societies work, and how they should facilitate those regime changes that are required to stop the spread of HIV. There are many of these lessons that are apparent, but they are so difficult to suggest, so culturally sensitive and often so politically incorrect, that few people push for their adoption, or think through what it would take to make them a reality.

Here is the beginning of a tentative list:

- In the context of hyper-epidemics, AIDS for the most part is heterosexually transmitted. AIDS is an indictment of male sexual behaviour in Africa. If AIDS were a crime, then men would be the perpetrators in the context of mature pandemics. The meanings attributed to and the signs and behaviours associated with African 'masculinity' are inimical to any constructive efforts to intervene in the spread of the pandemic in African communities. Profound cultural challenges and changes are required to address the politics of intimacy.
- Related to this, but going beyond the African continent, there are lessons to be learned regarding sexual networking, and on multiple concurrent partnering in particular. Early in the pandemic, behaviour change amongst gay men in the West as well as amongst Ugandans demonstrate that the lessons of AIDS can be heeded; sexual or other notions of 'culture' is not an untouchable fetish never to be challenged. This requires sustained and long-term thinking.
- AIDS has also demonstrated that transnational civil society can be an immensely powerful force. This kind of mobilisation has led to the changes made to the global intellectual property regime governing essential medications, and should be expanded to include other areas as well.
- Overseas development assistance is no substitute for home-grown economic growth and sound economic management with an emphasis on redistribution and justice. Donors are fickle and driven by political considerations that are not sustainable. In order for affected countries and communities to be self-sustaining, the global trade regime must change in order to free poor countries from the bonds of dependency, and to reduce poverty and marginalisation.
- AIDS is an extraordinary epidemic, and therefore it requires extraordinary thinkers and ideas. One example of such innovation is Parkhurst's and Whiteside's (2010) suggestion that a population-wide interruption of risk behaviour for a set period of time could reduce HIV incidence. Models estimate that up to half of all HIV acquisition arises from sex with an individual within the 'high viral load' first month after that person's own seroconversion. If one could get whole societies to either abstain from sex or only to have safe sex for one full month, then that could potentially create a feedback loop that will reduce the aggregate seroconversions in a specific community, lowering incidence levels. The policy implication of such a strategy could involve a 'safe sex/no sex' campaign in a cohesive population. In their article, Whiteside and Parkhurst refer to Ramadan, when

Muslims abstain from sex during daylight hours for a month, as evidence that people can reduce risky sexual behaviours over a set period of time.
- Elsewhere (Fourie 2006a) we have suggested that AIDS could assist traditional societies in particular in a move to secularisation, to question the more negative aspects of metaphysical moral scripts and superstition regarding not only AIDS, but other epidemics and society more generally. On this point, the unfortunate truth is that the converse can also happen: many African societies and governments are in fact becoming more and not less conservative and morally prescriptive as a response to the pandemic. However, an emphasis on constitutionalism, or enshrining secularism in a national constitution may in some instances protect against populist or politically regressive responses to AIDS (Ashforth 2005).
- We have also speculated that AIDS could mobilise a reconceptualisation of gender relations, and an 'AIDS feminism' (Fourie 2006b) that may transcend the place of women in vernacular societies, in particular. In a future scenario-building project to understand the future impact of AIDS in Africa (UNAIDS 2005), such reconceptualised gender relations are viewed as an example of new forms of social capital which can be activated in response to the pandemic.

Conclusion: the political imperative

The list above is only a start. There are many more lessons to be learnt from the AIDS pandemic – about how political scientific thinking can contribute, but also about what it means to be a caring society, about the relationship between men and women, about epidemiological exceptionalism, about the political perils of stigmatisation. Governments are only starting to explore the meaning of 'good AIDS governance' (Baldwin 2005, Strand 2007), and one prominent insight has been that what works in one context, could be entirely destructive in another.

These conversations about systemic, long-term change, adaptability and, ultimately, social resilience in the face of AIDS are difficult and often confronting to the mental maps and governance models that have come to be so closely associated with the pandemic. The political sciences can help to make sense of this, by broadening its focus towards more serious theorising of the pandemic.

The interdisciplinarity and intersubjectivity innate to resilience thinking can contribute to this, methodologically as well as theoretically. As quoted earlier, Holling *et al.* (2002, p. 5) emphasise that resilience thinking '... must of necessity transcend boundaries of scale and discipline. It must be capable of organising our understanding of economic, ecological and institutional systems'. Resilience thinking underlines change and uncertainty over time, and stresses the imperative for applied interdisciplinary knowledge in order to sustain systemic innovation.

Developing social resilience implies the identification and governance of not only the consequences of patterns of human behaviour, but also the identification and proactive management of the *systemic drivers/determinants* of that behaviour. In short, social resilience insists on vigilance and innovation regarding both the bio-natural ecosystem and the political and cultural institutions that determine how societies organise.

Methodologically, this is a tall order: it is indeed a challenge to identify all these factors, from so many different points of view, and within a long-wave timeframe. But this is the role of theory: to respect complexity and to simplify it, without rendering it simplistic. If the political sciences can step up to the task, it can help to build resilience in the face of wicked problems such as AIDS; it will also contribute to the resilience of political science itself.

Notes

1. Notable exceptions include the works of Altman (1986, 1994) and Bayer (1989).
2. As pointed out below and elsewhere (De Waal 2006 and Fourie 2009), given that over five million Africans are now on treatment, this threat has thus far proved to be empty. However, given recent shifts in multilateral and other public health funding and programmatic priorities, there is no guarantee that treatment will continue or that there will be new funds to continue the recent trajectory of treatment expansion.

References

Adger, W., 2000. Social and ecological resilience: are they related? *Progress in Human Geography*, 24 (3), 347–364.
Altman, D., 1986. *AIDS in the mind of America*. Garden City, NY: Anchor Press/Doubleday.
Altman, D., 1994. *Power and community: organizational and cultural responses to AIDS*. London: Taylor & Francis.
Ashforth, A., 2005. *Witchcraft, violence and democracy in South Africa*. Chicago: University of Chicago Press.
Baker, R., 2007. *Epidemic: the past, present and future of the diseases that made us*. London: Vision.
Baldwin, P., 2005. *Disease and democracy: the industrialized world faces AIDS*. Berkeley, CA: University of California Press.
Ball, P., 2004. *Critical mass: how one thing leads to another*. London: Arrow Books.
Barnes, E., 2005. *Diseases and human evolution*. Albuquerque, NM: University of New Mexico Press.
Barnett, T., 2006. A long-wave event. HIV/AIDS, politics, governance and 'security': sundering the intergenerational bond? *International Affairs*, 82 (2), 297–313.
Bayer, R., 1989. *Private acts, social consequences: AIDS and the politics of public health*. New York: The Free Press.
Bell, C., Devarajan, S., and Gersbach, H., 2006. The long-run economic costs of AIDS: a model with an application to South Africa. *World Bank Economic Review*, 20 (1), 55–89.
Cartwright, F. and Biddiss, M., 2006. *Disease & history*. Stroud: Sutton Publishing Ltd.
Chirambo, K., 2006. *Democratisation in the age of HIV/AIDS*. Pretoria: IDASA.
Cohn, S., 2007. After the Black Death: labour legislation and attitudes towards labour in late-medieval western Europe. *Economic History Review*, 60 (3), 457–485.
Colgan, J., Keohane, R., and Van de Graaf, T., 2011. Punctuated equilibrium in the energy regime complex. *The Review of International Organizations*. Available from: www.springerlink.com/content/g52862pp15572540 [accessed 26 July 2011].
Cooper, A. and Kirton, J., 2008. *Innovation in global health governance: critical cases*. Aldershot: Ashgate.
Crawford, D., 2007. *Deadly companions: how microbes shaped our history*. Oxford: OUP.
Diamond, J., 2005. *Collapse: how societies choose to fail or survive*. London: Allen Lane.
Easton, D., 1965. *A systems analysis of political life*. New York: Wiley.
Elbe, S., 2009. *Virus alert: security, governmentality and the AIDS Pandemic*. New York: Columbia University Press.
Epstein, H., 2007. *The invisible cure: africa, the west and the fight against AIDS*. London: Penguin.
Evans, R., 1988. Epidemics and revolutions: cholera in nineteenth-century Europe. *Past and Present*, no. 120, August, 123–146.
Ferguson, N., 2010. Complexity and collapse: empires on the edge of chaos. *Foreign Affairs*, 89 (2), 18–32.
Fourie, P., 2006a. For a secular response to AIDS. *Mail & Guardian*, 27 October.
Fourie, P., 2006b. After 25 years of AIDS holy cows in South Africa have to go. *Beeld*, 30 November.
Fourie, P., 2009. The relationship between the AIDS pandemic and state fragility. *In*: P. Fourie, S. Maclean and S. Brown, eds. *Health for some: the political economy of global health governance*. Basingstoke and New York: Palgrave Macmillan, 67–84.
Friedman, S. and Mottiar, S., 2005. A rewarding engagement? The treatment action campaign and the politics of HIV/AIDS. *Politics & Society*, 33 (4), 511–565.
Fukuyama, F., 2003. *Our posthuman future: consequences of the biotechnology revolution*. London: Profile Books.
Galaz, V., et al., eds., 2010. Governance, complexity and resilience. *Global Environmental Change* 20 (3), 363–368.

Gladwell, M., 2000. *The tipping point: how little things can make a big difference*. London: Abacus.

Hays, J., 2009. *The burdens of disease: epidemics and human response in western history*. New Brunswick: Rutgers University Press.

Holling, C., 2001. Understanding the complexity of economic, ecological, and social systems. *Ecosystems*, 4 (5), 390–405.

Holling, C. and Gunderson, L., 2002. Resilience and adaptive cycles. *In*: L. Gunderson and C. Holling, eds. *Panarchy: understanding transformations in human and natural systems*. Washington, DC: Island Press, 27–33.

Holling, C., Gunderson, L., and Ludwig, D., 2002. In quest of a theory of adaptive change. *In*: L. Gunderson and C. Holling, eds. *Panarchy: understanding transformations in human and natural systems*. Washington, DC: Island Press, 3–24.

Homer-Dixon, T., 2006. *The upside of down: catastrophe, creativity, and the renewal of civilisation*. London: Souvenir Press.

IRIN News. 2010. Lesotho-Swaziland: a customs union to prevent failed states, *IRIN News*, 18 August.

Kaiser Family Foundation, 2007. *The multisectoral impact of the HIV/AIDS epidemic – a primer*. Menlo Park, CA: KFF.

Lyman, P. and Wittels, S., 2010. No good deed goes unpunished: the unintended consequences of Washington's HIV/AIDS programs. *Foreign Affairs*, 89 (4), 74–84.

Marshall, N. and Marshall, P., 2007. Conceptualizing and operationalizing social resilience within commercial fisheries in northern Australia. *Ecology and Society*, 12 (1). Available from: http://www.ecologyandsociety.org/vol12/iss1/art1/ [accessed 12 August 2010].

McMichael, A., 2004. Environmental and social influences on emerging infectious diseases: past, present and future. *Philosophical Transactions: Biological Sciences*, 359 (1447), 1049–1058.

Over, M., 2009. Opportunities for presidential leadership on AIDS: from 'an emergency plan' to a sustainable policy. *Revue d'Economie du Développement* (1), Special issue on Health and Development 2 (5), 71–105.

Over, M., 2010. The global AIDS transition: a feasible objective for AIDS policy, online Centre for Global Development (CGD) essay, May. Available from: www.cgdev.org [accessed 15 August 2010].

Parkhurst, J. and Whiteside, A., 2010. Innovative response for preventing HIV transmission: the protective value of population-wide interruptions of risk activity. *The Southern African Journal of HIV Medicine*, 11 (1), 19–21.

Rostow, W., 1960. *The stages of economic growth: a non-communist manifesto*. Cambridge: CUP.

Seckinelgin, H., 2008. *International politics of HIV/AIDS – global disease, local pain*. Abingdon: Routledge.

Sidibé, M., Tanaka, S., and Buse, K., eds., 2010. Global health governance and the AIDS response, special edition of Global Health Governance. *The Scholarly Journal for the New Health Security Paradigm*, 4(1), 1–17.

Smith, A., 2010. Lesotho's people plead with South Africa to annex their troubled country. *The Observer*, 6 June.

Sontag, S., 2002. *Illness as metaphor and AIDS and its metaphors*. London: Penguin Books.

Sontag, S., 2003. *Regarding the pain of others*. New York: Picador/Farrar, Straus and Giroux.

Strand, P., 2007. Comparing AIDS governance: a research agenda on responses to the AIDS epidemic. *In*: N. Poku, A. Whiteside and B. Sandklaer, eds. *AIDS and governance*. Aldershot: Ashgate, 92–105.

Strand, P., et al., 2004. *HIV/AIDS and democratic governance in South Africa: illustrating the impact on electoral processes*. Pretoria: Institute for Democracy in South Africa.

Tainter, J., 2008. *The collapse of complex societies*. Cambridge: CUP.

Treichler, P., 1999. *How to have theory in an epidemic*. Durham: Duke University Press.

UNAIDS, 2005. *AIDS in africa: three scenarios to 2025*. Geneva: WHO.

UNAIDS, 2010. *Getting to zero: 2011–2015 strategy*. Geneva: WHO.

de Waal, A., 2006. *AIDS and power: why there is no political crisis – yet*. London: Zed Books.

de Waal, A. and Whiteside, A., 2006. AIDS: a Darwinian event? *In*: P. Denis and C. Becker, eds. *The HIV/AIDS epidemic in sub-saharan Africa in a historical perspective*. Louvain-la-Neuve: Academia-Bruylant, 57–72.

Walker, B. and Salt, D., 2006. *Resilience thinking: sustaining ecosystems and people in a changing world*. Washington, DC: Island Press.

Walker, B., *et al.*, 2006. A handful of heuristics and some propositions for understanding resilience in social-ecological systems. *Ecology and Society*, 11 (1), 1–15.

WHO, 2012. *International health regulations*. Geneva: WHO. Available from: http://www.who.int/topics/international_health_regulations/en/ [accessed 19 February 2012].

Wilson, M., 1995. Infectious diseases: an ecological perspective. *British Medical Journal*, 311 (7021), 1681–1684.

Index

Note: Page numbers in **bold** type refer to figures
Page numbers in *italic* type refer to *tables*
Page number followed by 'n' refer to notes

accidental infection 107–8
accountability 51–2; clientelistic 51
Act Up Paris 81
activism 3–5, 10, 19, 66, 74–84, 88; achievements 3–5, 109; campaigns/associations 76–84; homosexual 75–81; political achievements 3–5; and social movements 19
Adger, W. 133
Africa 18–19, 24–5; accountability 51–2; AIDS constituency natures 55–7, *56–7*; electoral choice determinants 50; employee infection/mortality 18; and military 116–22; Renaissance 25; South 30–47; and state health partnerships 17–18, *see also* public opinion survey
African National Congress (ANC) 32
Afrobarometer 51–2, 91
AIDS: The Greatest Leadership Challenge (EC) 115
AIDS and the Military (UNAIDS) 118
AIDS Prevention and Support Group (GAPA) 66
AIDS Reference and Treatment Centre (Brazil/S America) 66
AIDS Security and Conflict Initiative (ASCI) 124
AIDS, Security and the Military in Africa (Whiteside *et al*) 119
AIDS-Hilfe Schweiz (Swiss Help Against AIDS) 76
AIDS2031 Report 6
Aizhixing Legal AID Centre 106–7
Albertyn, C. 32
Allen, T.: and Heald, S. 17
Altman, D. 17, 65, 118, 123; and Buse, K. 1–14
Anan, K. 115
And the Band Played on (Shilts) 7
Anderson, R. 136
Angels in America (Kushner) 8
anonymous testing 77

anti-retroviral therapies/treatments (ARV/Ts) 21, 54, 87, 95, 124; free 37, 42, 93–4
antibiotics/vaccines 134
apartheid 25
Asia Catalyst 103–5
Asia Pacific Ministerial Meeting on HIV/AIDS 115
Asia-Pacific Consultation on HIV and Sex Work 104
Asia-Pacific Network of Sex Workers (APNSW) 104–5

Baker, R. 134
Ball, P. 131
Barnett, T.: and Prins, G. 120, 123
Barrett, E. 32
Becker, J.: *et al* 119
Beja, J. 109
Bill and Melinda Gates Foundation 10, 116
biopower 60–2
Birth of Biopolitics, The (Foucault) 61
Black Death 134–6
Black Sash 32
Blair, A. 5
blood donors 101
Bratton, M. 50–1, 55–6
Brazil 60–73; capacity-building 60–70; governmentality 60–2, 69–70; National STD/AIDS programme 60, 66; networks 62–5; Universal Healthcare System (SUS) 65; vulnerability 60–5
Brazilian Harm Reducers Association (ABORDA) 70
Brazilian Interdisciplinary AIDS Association (ABIA) 66
Brazilian Prostitutes Network 67, 70
Bretton-Woods 64
BRICS states (Brazil/Russia/India/China/S Africa) 6, 9
Bright Futures Group 90
Broqua, C. 81
Buckley, W. 10
Buse, K.: and Altman, D. 1–14

INDEX

Bush, George W. 4–7, 115

Câmara da Silva, C. 66
Campbell, C. 63
capacity-building (CICT) 60–70, see also Brazil
Cardoso, F. 69–70
Central Intelligence Agency (CIA) 117
Cernea, M. 67
Chambre, S. 62–3
Chattopadhyay, R.: and Duflo, E. 32
China 99–112; Access to Medicines Research Group 108; accidental infection compensation 107–8; AIDS policy background 100–1; Central Party School 107; discrimination protection 106–7; global governance response innovations 101–2; HIV/AIDS Information Network/Control Programme 105, 108; medicine access 108; Open Door Policy 102; sex worker representation and protection 104–5; State Council AIDS Working Committee 101; State Intellectual Property Office (SIPO) 108; transnational connections/civil society organization (TNCS) 102–8
China Cares 106
China Centre for Disease Control (CDC) 101
China Global Fund Watch 103, 106
Chinese People's Political Consultative Congress 108
Chirac, J. 5
cholera 134
church membership 4; leadership 88
civil death concept 66
civil rights 19
civil society organizations (CSOs) 17–18
class/gender/race issues 18, 38, 44
Cold War 21, 114
Collapse: How Societies Chose to Fail or Survive (Diamond) 133
Collapse of Complex Societies, The (Tainter) 133
collectivism 93
Collor, F. 66
colonialism 20
commercial sex 6, see also sex workers
Comprehensive Poverty Reduction and Growth Strategy 94
condom use promotion 9, 77, 101
Confucian belief systems 101, 104
contagion: and morality 92
Cooper, A.: and Kirton, J. 135
Coordination Homosexuelle Suisse (CHOSE) 75–6
Council on Foreign Relations report (Garrett) 119

Critical Mass (Ball) 131
Cruikshank, B. 70
culture, role 8; identities and ideologies 17

Daniel, H. 66
death: civil concept 66
Declaration of Commitment on HIV/AIDS (UNGASS) 115
Defense Department (US) 117; HIV/AIDS Prevention Programme (DHAAP) 121–2
Dehesa, R. de la: and Mukherjea, A. 60–73
denialism 19–20
Deutsche Aids-Hilfe 77
Diamond, J. 133
Diamond, L. 44
Dionne, K. 24, 38
disciplinarity 15
discrimination 92; employment/education 106–7; and legal protection 19, 106–7; non 102
donors and funders 20, 94, 101; blood 101; patronage network 95–6; treatment programmes 95
drug users 92; illicit 92, 100; injecting (IDUs) 4–6, 66, 88–9, 91–4, 100; methadone maintenance programmes 95
drugs: approval 19; donations 4
Duflo, E.: and Chattopadhyay, R. 32
Duyvendak, J. 76

Eade, D. 65
Eberstadt, N. 118
Economic Commission (EC): African Development Forum 115
Economist 10
Elbe, S. 17, 21, 118–19, 122–3
Elias, N. 75
ELISA test 78
Enlightenment 135
Epstein, H. 8
Epstein, S. 63, 67
Evolutionary Theory 129
exceptionalism 1, 75, 81

Fala Mulher da Vida 67
Family Watch International 9
Farmer, P. 65
Federal Office of Public Health (FOPH) 76, 79–80
feedback loops 131
feminist movements 88, 139
Ferguson, N. 130
feudalism 135
Fillieule, O.: and Voegtli, M. 74–86
finance issues 8; donors and funders 20
Fleury, S. 65
Florini, A.: and Simmons, P. 104

INDEX

Follér, M.: and Fourie, P. 9, 128–42
Foucault, M. 60–1, 71n, 134–6
Fourie, P.: and Follér, M. 9, 128–42
Freedom House 89
Frolic, B. 103
funders *see* donors and funders

G-8 summits 5–6; Gleneagles (2005) 5
G-20 summits 6
Galaz, V.: *et al* 133
Galvao, J. 68
Garrett, L. 119
Gay Identity 75
gay/lesbian/bisexual/transgender (GLBT) 19, 62, 88; Brazilian Association (ABGLT) 69; and gender role changes 20
gender/race/class issues 18, 38, 44
General Assembly 3
General Plan to Reform the State Apparatus (Brazil) 69
Germ Theory 134
Gladwell, M. 131
Global Business Coalition on AIDS 102
Global Fund to Fight AIDS: country coordinating mechanism (CCM) 100, 105; election controversy 105–6; Tuberculosis and Malaria 3–4, 10, 18, 94–5, 101, 108
Global Infectious Disease Threat and Implications (NIC) 117–19, 122
Global Network of People Living with HIV and AIDS (GNP+) 102
Global Network of Sex Work Projects 105
Global Program on AIDS 30
Gore, A. 115
governance 23–5; African 17, 48–58; and civil conflict 23–5; civil society inclusion/participation 105–6; good practices 128, 139; research agenda 23; structures 132–3
governmentality 60–2, 69–70; and biopower 60–2; neo-liberal 61, 71
Greater Involvement of People with AIDS initiative (GIPA) 89–91
Grebe, E. 63
Grupo Gay da Bahia movement 66
Guehenno, J-M. 121
Gunderson, L.: and Holling, C. 131
Guta, A.: *et al* 63

haemophiliacs 19
Heald, S.: and Allen, T. 17
health 82; biomedical agendas 93; education 95; insurance 77; life expectancy 82; medicine access 108; and poverty 130; public approach 61, 95, *see also* FOPH
Highly Active Antiretroviral Therapy (HAART) 75, 79–83
HIV/AIDS Alliance 106

Hogan, B. 33
Holbrooke, R. 114–16, 123
Holling, C.: *et al* 130, 133, 139; and Gunderson, L. 131
Homer-Dixon, T. 133
homophobia 69
homosexuality 9, 19, 100; and activism 75–81; anti attitudes 88; and associative space 74–85; (MSMs) 89, 100–5
Hudson, R. 134
human rights 4–6, 48, 93, 100, 106–7; campaigners 4, 32; organizations 103
hyper-epidemics 128–42; deep and systemic change 136–9; impacts 128–36; long-wave nature 136–7; major aspects 16; political change in history 133–6; political imperative 139; recommendations 136; scientific foundations 130–3; short-termism 137; and social resilience 128–39
hypocrisy 8

identity 88; differences (competing/collective) 91–2
infection: accidental 107–8; vulnerability 6
Institute of Religious Studies 66–7; Prostitution and Human Rights programme 66–7
institution-building 64
insurance coverage 77; health 77
intellectual property (IP) law 21
Inter Agency Standing Committee 116
International AIDS Conference 2, 25; Asia and Pacific 3
International AIDS Society (IAS) 1–3, 10
International Centre for Technical Cooperation on HIV/AIDS (Brazil) 60
International Council of AIDS Service Organizations 10, 106
international development 19–21
International Health Regulations 135
International Labour Organization (ILO) 102; Code of Practice on HIV/AIDS and the World of Work 106
international organizations (IOs) 18
International Relations in the New Century 114
International Republican Institute (IRI) 105–6
interstitial elites 20–1
IRIN News 129
isolationism 100–2

Justesen, M. 56

Kaiser Family Foundation 96
Kaplan, R. 7
Kaufman, J. 99–112

INDEX

Keck, M.: and Sikkink, K. 63, 103, 107
Kirton, J.: and Cooper, A. 135
Klerk, F.W. de 25
Korekata AIDS Law Centre 107
Kramer, L. 8
Kushner, T. 8

Lasswell, H. 2
lesbians 19, see also GLBT
Leyi (Shanghai) 107
Lieberman, E. 17, 30–47, 50
life expectancy 48
low-and-middle income countries (LMIC) 102
Lowicki-Zucca, M.: et al 119
Lula, L. 70
Lush, L.: and Parkhurst, J. 17

McInnes, C. 22, 119–20; and Rushton, S. 123
McMichael, A. 135
Make Poverty History movement 5
malaria 134; and tuberculosis 3–4, 10, 18, 94–5, 101, 108, see also Global Fund
Mandela, N. 25
Mansbridge, J. 31
Marshall, N.: and Marshall, P. 133
Mattes, R. 51, 57
Mbeki, President Thabo 2, 19, 25
MDGs 5, 9; as global operating development framework 5
Medecins Sans Frontiers (MSF) 19
men who have sex with men (MSMs) 66, 69, 91; behaviour 103–5
Merson, M. 30
methadone maintenance programmes 95
military prevalence 21–3; and African epidemics 116–22, *117*; AIDS hypothesis 113–27; priority justification 114; securitization 114–24, see also security
Millennium Development Goals (MDG) 5, 9, 58
mobilization 87–98; competing/collective identities 91–2; differences 91–6; economic and external structures 93–6; lessons 87–8; movements/goals 90–1; political culture 93–6; Zambia/Vietnam country cases and methodology 88–90
morality 4, 101; and authority of law 106–7; and contagion 92
mortality 52–4, 62
Most Important Problem (MIP) 52–4
Motsoaledi, A. 33
Mukherjea, A.: and de la Dehesa, R. 60–73
multi-national corporations (MNCs) 17, 21
multiplacadores (multiplying agents, Brazil) 66
Museveni, Y. 17, 24

National AIDS Commission (Brazil) 66
National Intelligence Council (NIC) 117–18, 122
National Meetings of AIDS NGOs (ENONGS) (Brazil) 66
National STD/AIDS Programme (Brazil) 60, 66; First AIDS and STD Control project (AIDS I) 68; Maria Sem Vergonha Project 70; NGO Articulation Unit 66–8; Previna-high risk group prevention project 66–7, 70; Roda Brasil Project 70; SOMOS Project 69–70; Tulipa Project 70
National Transvestites and Transexual Articulation (ANTRA) 70
nationalism 100
needle usage 6, see also drug users
neoliberalism 61, 71
Network for Zambian People Living with HIV/AIDS (NZP+) 90–3
New Public Management (NPM) 79
New Yorker 8
non-governmental organizations (NGOs) 17–18, 23, 106; work (medical/political/humanitarian etc) 20
Normal Heart, The (Kramer) 8

Observer 129
O'Keefe, M. 113–27
one-size-fits-all prevention strategy 17
Ostergard, R. 22
Over, M. 138

Pact 106
Parker, R. 10
Parkhurst, J.: and Lush, L. 17; and Whiteside, A. 138
pathogens 135–6
Pathologies of Power (Farmer) 65
patrimonialism 50
Patterson, A.: and Stephens, D. 87–98
Patton, C. 63
Paxton, N. 7–9, 15–29
people living with HIV and AIDS (PLWHA) 18–19, 24, 101; and secondary marginalization 19
people living with HIV (PLHIVs) 87–96
Pimenta, C.: et al 67
Piot, P. 115
Pitkin, H. 31–2
pluralism 96
Poggione, S. 32
policy networks 18
political science 7–8; as art 10–11; critical analysis 15–29; failure 7–8; global and comparative health 16; governance 23–5; HIV epidemic major aspects 16; international development 19–21; and

INDEX

rights 19; security 21–3; social movements/activism 19; state partnerships for health/performance 16–18
Posner, D. 50
poverty 48, 94; and health 130; reduction 93
pre-employment/recruitment testing 121
President's (US) Emergency Plan for AIDS Relief (PEPFAR) 7, 94–6, 115
pricing, tiered 4
Prins, G.: and Barnett, T. 120, 123
Prostitution and Civil Rights programme (Brazil) 67
public opinion survey 48–59; accountability 51–2; AIDS constituency natures 52, 55–7, 56–7; AIDS response in Africa 48–58; conditions 49; description 52–7; electoral choice determinants 50; and HIV prevalence link 55; inclusion determinants 56–7, 57; and objective data link 52–5, 53–4
Public-Private Partnerships (PPPs) 23
Punctuated Equilibrium Theory 129
Putzel, J. 24–5

race/class/gender issues 18, 44; categories 38, see also South Africa
Ratti, A. 76–7
Raviglione, M.: and Smith, I. 30
Reidener, H. 76
religion 8, 96; Christian 9, 135; Islamic 9
research agenda 8–10; and care 19
resilience, social 128–39; adaptive cycle 132; principles 132–3; scientific foundations 130–3; thinking 130–3, 137–9; understanding 129–33, see also hyper-epidemics
Resolution 1308 (UN 2000) 116–18, 123
rights: civil 19; human 106; and political science 19
rights-holders 21
Rochefoucauld, F. de la 8
Rosen, S. 22
Rosenbrock, R.: et al 79
Rushton, S.: and McInnes, C. 123

Sabatier, P. 9
safe sex education 9; and practices 61–3
SAHARA Conference (South Africa) 3
Salt, D.: and Walker, B. 130–3
Sato, A. 124
Sawicki, F.: and Siméant, J. 84
Schwindt-Bayer, L. 32
security 21–3, 130, 136; agenda evidence 117–18; and evidence gap 120–2; military AIDS hypothesis 113–24; political birth and military 114–16; revisionists 119–20, 124;
and securitization 114–24; and war conduct (militarising) 22–3
Setbon, M. 75
sex: commercial 6; men with men (MSMs) 66, 69, 91, 103–5; safe (education) 9, 61–3
sex workers 6, 61–4, 67, 76, 88–9, 91–2, 100; and capacity-building programmes 64; networks and projects 104–5; as peer educators 67; representation and protection (China) 104–5
sexual rights 6, see also activism
Shilts, R. 7
Sidibé, M. 101
Sikkink, K.: and Keck, M. 63, 103, 107
Silva Leite, G. 67
Siméant, J.: and Sawicki, F. 84
Simmons, P.: and Florini, A. 104
Singer, P. 118–19
smallpox 134
Smith, I.: and Raviglione, M. 30
Smith, J.: and Whiteside, A. 124
social movements: and activism 19
social resilience 128–39
social workers 76; and drug users 76
socio-economic issues 18
soft power approach 103–4
Somaini, B. 76
Sontag, S. 136
South Africa 30–47; AIDS policy 30–45; analysis 39–44; councillor characteristics (race/gender) 38–9, 38; councillor descriptive statistics 39–44, 40; councillor policy preferences, measurement/distribution 35–8, 35–6; *Democracy in South Africa* (attitudes/opinions) questionnaire 34–44; drug testing/free provision 36–7, 42–4; gender and race differences 32–3, 39–44, 41–3; health ministers 33; incarceration 42; research design 33–45; Treatment Action Campaign 63
Specter, M. 8
Spiegel, P. 121
Staub, R. 76–7
Stephens, D.: and Patterson, A. 87–98
stigmatization 92, 100
STOP AIDS campaign 78
Strand, P. 24, 48–59
Strike Hard campaigns 104
surveillance 135
Swiss AIDS Federation (SAF). creation 76–85
Swiss Organization of Homophiles (SOH) 75–6
Switzerland 74–86; Association changes/membership withdrawal 78–9; cantonal level financing pattern changes 81–4, 83;

INDEX

Confederation financing 79–84, 80; exceptionalism phase 75, 81; and HAART introduction 75, 79–83; initial response formation 75–9; mobilization process 84–5; normalization of HIV/AIDS 75, 79–84; transformation effects 80–1; treatment impacts 81–2; volunteer withdrawals 83–4
Systems Theory 129

Tages Anzeiger 78
Tainter, J. 133
testing 77; anonymous 77; pre-employment/recruitment 121
Thinking Politically initiative 1, 7–8, 11
Thomas, S.: and Welch, S. 32
Tipping Point, The (Gladwell) 131
tokenism 91
tradition, role 8
transnational corporations (TNCs) 101–8
Treatment Action Campaign (TAC) 19, 25, 56, 88, 102, 108
Treichler, P. 63
Tshabalala-Msimang, M. 33
tuberculosis (TB): control program 30; drug-resistant forms 37; epidemic 31–5, 42–4; and malaria 3–4, 10, 18, 94–5, 101, 108; risk perceptions 35–8, *see also* Global Fund
typhus 134

Ulmann, M. 76
UNITAID 10, 101
United Nations Development Programme (UNDP) 89, 107
United Nations General Assembly special session (UNGASS) 101–2, 115
United Nations HIV/AIDS Programme (UNAIDS) 1–4, 10, 18, 48, 100–1, 104–9, 115–23
United Nations Security Council (UNSC) 3–5, 22, 114–16, 121–3; Resolution 1308 (2000) 116–18, 123
United Nations (UN) 1–5, 102, 109, 121; Agenda (21) 64; Declaration 48; Environment and Development Conference (1992) 64; Human Rights and HIV 106; Office for Coordination of Humanitarian Affairs 129; Treaty on Economic, Social and Cultural Rights 106
Upside of Down, The (Homer-Dixon) 133

vaccines 134
victim blaming 101
Vietnam 87–98; AIDS mobilization 88–96; cases and methodology 88–90; competing/collective identities 91–2; difference epidemics 91; economic and external structures 93–6; political culture 93–6; Zambia comparison 87–96
Vietnam National Network of People Living with HIV/AIDS (VNP+) 90
Vietnam Positive Women's Network (VPWN) 90
violence: sexual 22, 63
Voegtli, M.: and Fillieule, O. 74–86
vulnerability 6, 60–5; infection 6; populations 60–5, *see also* Brazil

Waal, A. de 23, 49, 122
Walker, B.: and Salt, D. 130–3
Welch, S.: and Thomas, S. 32
Wen Jibao 107
Whiteside, A. 20; *et al* 119; and Parkhurst, J. 138; and Smith, J. 124
Wilson, M. 135
Wilson, S. 103
Women's League 32
World AIDS Day 90–2
World Bank 64–70, 137; International Forum on Capacity-Building of Southern NGOs 68; NGO Committee 67–8; Operational Manual Statement 67
World Health Organization (WHO) 18, 131, 135; Global programme on AIDS 18
World Trade Organization (WTO) 21, 108; Doha Declaration 21, 108; and public health 9, 21; trade-related aspects of intellectual property (TRIPS) 108

Youde, J. 17–19

Zambia 87–98; AIDS mobilization 88–96; country case comparison 87–96, *see also* Vietnam
Zambia Network of Religious Leaders Living with/Personally Affected by HIV/AIDS (ZANERELA+) 90–3
Zambian Interfaith Networking Group on HIV/AIDS (ZINGO) 90–3
Zurich: gay liberation group (HAZ) 76; leather association 76